Basics of Public Health Core Competencies

Larry Holmes, Jr., PhD, DrPH

Clinical Epidemiologist
Alfred I. duPont Hospital for Children
Wilmington, Delaware

Head, Molecular Epidemiology Laboratory
Nemours Center for Childhood Cancer Research
Wilmington, Delaware

Adjunct Associate Professor
University of Delaware
Dover, Delaware

JONES AND BARTLETT PUBLISHERS
Sudbury, Massachusetts
BOSTON   TORONTO   LONDON   SINGAPORE

World Headquarters

Jones and Bartlett Publishers
40 Tall Pine Drive
Sudbury, MA 01776
978-443-5000
info@jbpub.com
www.jbpub.com

Jones and Bartlett Publishers
Canada
6339 Ormindale Way
Mississauga, Ontario L5V 1J2
Canada

Jones and Bartlett Publishers
International
Barb House, Barb Mews
London W6 7PA
United Kingdom

Jones and Bartlett's books and products are available through most bookstores and online booksellers. To contact Jones and Bartlett Publishers directly, call 800-832-0034, fax 978-443-8000, or visit our website www.jbpub.com.

Substantial discounts on bulk quantities of Jones and Bartlett's publications are available to corporations, professional associations, and other qualified organizations. For details and specific discount information, contact the special sales department at Jones and Bartlett via the above contact information or send an email to specialsales@jbpub.com.

This publication is designed to provide accurate and authoritative information in regard to the Subject Matter covered. It is sold with the understanding that the publisher is not engaged in rendering legal, accounting, or other professional service. If legal advice or other expert assistance is required, the service of a competent professional person should be sought.

Production Credits

Publisher: Michael Brown
Production Director: Amy Rose
Associate Editor: Katey Birtcher
Editorial Assistant: Catie Heverling
Production Editor: Tracey Chapman
Marketing Manager: Sophie Fleck
Manufacturing and Inventory Control Supervisor: Amy Bacus
Composition: Arlene Apone
Illustrator: Accurate Artists, Inc.
Cover Design: Brian Moore
Printing and Binding: Malloy, Inc.
Cover Printing: Malloy, Inc.

Library of Congress Cataloging-in-Publication Data

Holmes, Larry, 1960-
    Basics of public health core competencies / Larry Holmes Jr.
        p. ; cm.
    Includes bibliographical references and index.
    ISBN-13: 978-0-7637-6537-8 (pbk.)
    ISBN-10: 0-7637-6537-6 (pbk.)
    1. Public health. I. Title.
    [DNLM: 1. Public Health—methods. 2. Biometry—methods. 3. Epidemiologic Methods. 4. Professional Competence. WA 100 H751b 2009]
    RA425.H582 2009
    362.1—dc22
                                                    2008026277

6048

Printed in the United States of America
12 11 10 09 08   10 9 8 7 6 5 4 3 2 1

DEDICATION

In memory of my grandmother (Nkoyo Attah), grandfather (Duke Holmes), father (Morrison Holmes), and Laura Krueger, Elton Krueger, and Willie Kolwes of Brenham, Texas, whose lives and dedication to family values reflect true leadership in public health. I offer my thanks for their perpetual application of the fundamental principles of family/socioeconomic support systems in enabling healthful lifestyles and outcomes.

In a very special way, to the memory of my mom (Koko), who passed away during the gestation period of this book.

CONTENTS

Introduction: Public Health Science: Principles and Practice   xxiii

Chapter 1: Principles and Methods of Biostatistics   1

FOREWORD

Public health—the science and art of disease prevention and health promotion—remains central to the advances of medical and health sciences in ameliorating the health of the population. The contribution of public health to the health of the U.S. population has been remarkable in the 21st century, and it continues to be so as public health confronts emerging challenges due to the aging U.S. population, climate changes, global warming, bioterrorism, and emerging pathogenic microbes. Remarkably, the epidemiologic transition from infectious diseases as the leading cause of mortality in the 1900s to chronic diseases today came as a result of persistent immunization, the reduction in vaccine-preventable diseases, and improvements in sanitation and nutrition—even before the streptomycin trials in *mycobacterium tuberculae* in 1947—thanks to public health contributions. Illustratively, public health achievements in the 21st century are viewed in light of their contributions to motor vehicle safety, safer workplaces, infectious disease control, decline in coronary artery disease and stroke mortality, safer and healthier food, healthier mothers and babies, family planning, fluoridation of drinking water, vaccination, and recognition of tobacco as a health hazard.

The scope of public health is broad and reflects what we, as a society, do collectively to ensure the conditions necessary for people to remain healthy. Within this scope, the framework for public health performance recommends the collaboration between governmental agencies (federal, state, and local), public and private sectors, and the communities. The Institute of Medicine, in its 1988 response to "public health in disarray," clearly described the core functions of public health as (1) assessment, (2) policy development, and (3) assurance. The process upon which public health carries out these functions requires the integration of its core functions into the essential public health services, namely, (1) health services monitoring and identification of community health needs; (2) diagnoses and investigation of health problems and health hazards in the community; (3) informing, educating, and empowering people about health issues; (4) mobilizing community partnerships to identify and solve health problems; (5) enforcing laws and regulations that protect and ensure safety; (6) linking people with needed personal health services and ensuring the provision of health care when otherwise unavailable; (7) ensuring a competent public health and personal healthcare workforce; (8) evaluating effectiveness, accessibility, and quality of personal and population-based health services; and (9) researching new insights and innovative solutions to health problems.

The training of public health professionals to address the essential public health services requires a curriculum that integrates the core functions of public health into the core disciplines of public health, mainly (1) epidemiology, (2) biostatistics, (3) behavioral and social sciences, (4) environmental sciences, and (5) management and policy sciences. The knowledge of these areas and the application of cross-cutting core competencies (such as communication and informatics, diversity and culture, animal control, public health biology and pathology, professionalism, programs planning, and systems thinking) serve to provide the graduates of public health programs with the preparation (knowledge and skills) needed to succeed in this field today.

The author of and the contributors to this text, *Basics of Public Health Core Competencies,* have presented—in a simplified and concise manner—an introduction to public health as public health principles and practice, which is rarely presented in graduate programs, and have discussed the mission, goal, core functions, history, and challenges of public health. Whereas graduates of public health tend to focus on a set module or discipline, in spite of our recommendation of the broad knowledge of the public health core disciplines, this approach has made it possible for graduates and potential graduates of public health to acquire competency in these core areas. I hope that this work will point readers in a direction that will stimulate their appetites to learn more about the assessment of health issues in the population, about making sense of data, about the role of behavior in health, about the impact of environment on health as well as environmental justice, and about policy development in the management of public health services. If you believe that all books are perspectives, then no book, no matter the volume, will be able to present all the subject matter of any given field.

This book, which presents the core competencies as learning objectives, should serve to remind the faculty at the various schools of public health in the nation of what students are expected to acquire in terms of knowledge, attitudes, and skills prior to joining the public health workforce. Therefore, it is with great optimism that I recommend this book, with the hope that knowledge gained from a simplified text of this nature will inform quality performance and evidence-based public health as well as systems thinking in public health program development, conduct, and evaluation.

James Harlan Steele, DVM, MPH
Retired U.S. Assistant Surgeon General
Professor Emeritus, University of Texas
Health Sciences Center at Houston
School of Public Health
Houston, Texas

ACKNOWLEDGMENTS

Public health is an interdisciplinary science, requiring many subspecialties in its approach to disease prevention and health promotion. This book, *Basics of Public Health Core Competencies,* would never have been prepared without contributions from my colleagues from the various disciplines that sustain essential public health functions and research infrastructures.

This book has been written to aid in the understanding of the core competencies in public health. Schools of public health had traditionally prepared students to focus on their module or discipline with very little exposure to mastery in the five core disciplines: epidemiology, biostatistics, social and behavioral sciences, environmental sciences, and health policy and management sciences. Realistically, graduate programs are designed to create a focus, thus gearing toward specialized knowledge. However, a broad knowledge of these core disciplines requires not only introductory courses in these core areas but some level of formation and application of these concepts in the real world. With this gap in mind, this book has made it possible for graduates of public health programs to acquire some mastery in these core areas and the cross-cutting areas (communications and informatics, diversity and culture, leadership, public health biology, professionalism, programs planning, and systems thinking).

Many sources of information were consulted during the gestational period of this text. I am very grateful to all authors whose works we have consulted prior to the preparation of this book. I sincerely appreciate the knowledge and information gained from your intense and meaningful contributions to the field of public health. However, if you feel you have not been adequately acknowledged, I am willing to do so at the first opportunity.

I am indebted to my colleagues at the Texas Medical Center, who provided instant assistance when required to assemble research materials for the many sections in this book that required extra-intense review. It will be impossible to list names. I acknowledge, with thanks, your contributions.

I owe the chapters on basic sciences of public health to the experience gained from teaching graduate students in Texas and medical students in the Caribbean over the many years of my teaching career and, more recently, teaching surgical residents and postdoctoral research fellows in

Wilmington, Delaware. Because teaching is a learning experience, I have learned by teaching epidemiology and biostatistics in these settings. I hope this experience reflects the information provided in these two chapters.

I am indebted to my parents (deceased), uncles, and aunts for never asking me not to ask them "Why?" I am grateful to Jenni, my spouse and gatekeeper for our kids Maddy, MacKenzie, and Landon, and their grandparents, Dalton and Sue, for their patience and unconditional acceptance even when I avoided contact with them and turned to the computer in order to complete a sentence or section of this text. Likewise, I am sincerely and deeply grateful to my siblings and cousins for their encouragement—Victor, Paul, Brian, Ann, Julie, Nkoyo, Glory, Francis (deceased), Agnes, Charles, Ekaete (deceased), etc.

Public health is not an exact science. We have consulted with sources of information judged to be valid during the period of the preparation of this text. However, information presented today is subject to change as new information becomes available tomorrow. Therefore, readers are required to consult with similar sources for the confirmation of information provided here.

Finally, I am grateful to Michael Brown, Katey Birtcher, Tracey Chapman, and the staff at Jones and Bartlett for their enthusiasm and constant support.

CONTRIBUTORS

FOREWORD

James H. Steele, DVM, MPH
Retired U.S. Assistant Surgeon General
Professor Emeritus
University of Texas, School of Public Health
Houston, Texas

AUTHOR

Larry Holmes, Jr., PhD, DrPH
Clinical Epidemiologist
Alfred I. duPont Hospital for Children
Wilmington, Delaware

Head, Molecular Epidemiology Laboratory
Nemours Center for Childhood Cancer Research
Wilmington, Delaware

Adjunct Associate Professor
University of Delaware
Dover, Delaware

CONTRIBUTORS

John Balogun, MD, MPH
Disease Control and Preventive Health Services
University of Texas, School of Public Health
Houston, Texas

Joan Nwuli, JD
Health Policy and Management Sciences
Nwuli & Associates Law Firm
Houston, Texas

Gbade Ogungbade, DVM, PhD
Health Services and Health Policy and Management Sciences
Population Health Research Institute
Houston, Texas

Jennifer Thompson, MS, MA, MPH
Environmental Sciences
Harris County, Texas

Doriel D. Ward, PhD, MPH
Health Policy and Management Sciences and Behavioral Sciences
University of Texas, MD Anderson Cancer Center
Houston, Texas

ABOUT THE AUTHOR

Larry Holmes, Jr., PhD, DrPH, has more than nine years of experience as a reviewer of the U.S. Medical Licensing Examination (USMLE) questions (1994–2003). During this period, he taught quantitative medicine (epidemiology, biostatistics) among other courses and was responsible for both the summative and formative examination preparation materials for the medical schools in the Caribbean.

At the International University of the Health Sciences (IUHS) in St. Kitts, Holmes directed the assessment for the basic medical sciences and clinical correlates and managed more than 18,000 questions in the examination bank. He was responsible for preparing the summative examination of 350 questions for every organ-system in the USMLE learning objectives, and these examinations were offered every three months at IUHS. Holmes also wrote review questions for immunology and infectious diseases, quantitative medicine (epidemiology and biostatistics), preventive medicine, behavioral sciences, geriatrics, and pharmacology. In addition, Dr. Holmes was responsible for the development of the dual-pathway in medical education at IUHS, which involved the merging of the traditional approach to medical education with problem-based learning. He is very experienced in evaluating curriculum and determining the level of information necessary to meet the curriculum requirements. He has reflected this experience in his interpretation of the core competencies with respect to knowledge, skills, and attitude.

Holmes is currently a clinical epidemiologist at the Alfred I. duPont Hospital for Children in Wilmington, Delaware, where he oversees the clinical research methodology (modern epidemiology and biostatistics) research and education program for postdoctoral research fellows and surgical residents. He also heads the molecular epidemiology laboratory at the Nemours Center for Childhood Cancer Research. Holmes is a published primary or senior author in many peer-reviewed scientific journals, a reviewer for scientific journals including *Military Medicine* and *AIDS Care*, and a member of the American College of Epidemiology.

PREFACE

Public health can be defined as what we as a society can do to remain healthy. This broad notion of public health is indicative of the shared responsibility of the governmental agencies, public and private sectors, and the community in meeting the demands of the core functions of public health, namely, assessment, policy, and assurance. These core functions are fused into the essential public health services: (1) health services monitoring and identification of community health needs; (2) diagnoses and investigation of health problems and health hazards in the community; (3) informing, educating, and empowering people about health issues; (4) mobilizing community partnerships to identify and solve health problems; (5) enforcing laws and regulations that protect and ensure safety; (6) linking people with needed personal health services and ensuring the provision of health care when otherwise unavailable; (7) ensuring a competent public health and personal healthcare workforce; (8) evaluating effectiveness, accessibility, and quality of personal and population-based health services; and (9) researching new insights and innovative solutions to health problems.

The core functions of public health and the essential public health services serve as the reference point for the core competencies and cross-cutting areas in public health. The competencies in these core areas are indicative of the broad knowledge of public health in fulfilling its substance as declared by the Institute of Medicine in *The Future of Public Health: Disease Control Prevention and Health Promotion*. The core competencies simply set the path regarding the volume of knowledge, attitude, and skills required of graduates of public health in delivering public health direct services, research, and teaching.

There is a need to standardize these core disciplines in terms of the core competencies in order to administer an examination that will fairly test knowledge and performance in these core competencies and their cross-cutting areas. Using the core disciplines in public health and the cross-cutting areas (professionalism, leadership, systems thinking, program planning, diversity and culture, and public health biology), we reviewed public health knowledge and practice with the intent to provide candidates with the information needed to acquire public health competencies and obtain a high yield in the National Public Health Certification Examination.

This book is not a substitute for the recommended textbooks used in these various public health disciplines. To benefit from this book, graduates of public health are expected to have had a good exposure to these core disciplines prior to graduation. However, if less time was dedicated to these areas, readers will find this book useful, although not exhaustive. In this book we have tried to present the core competencies as the learning objectives for each of the chapters. To some, these learning objectives may appear novel, but this should not be the case since we utilized the American Society for Public Health (ASPH) guidelines available to Schools of Public Health in coding these learning objectives. For example, PHCC.1.3 refers to "Public Health Core Competencies, Biostatistics: Descriptive Techniques in Summarizing Public Health Data." Materials are presented throughout the chapter to reflect the depth of knowledge required to meet the objectives, as well as vignettes to illustrate the application of concept to the "real-world" situation.

The Introduction addresses the idea of public health and the mission, substance, and goal of public health. A brief history is offered to illustrate the role of public health in the epidemiologic transition from infectious diseases to chronic diseases. The achievements of public health during the 21st century are presented as well as the current challenges of the field. Chapter 1 presents biostatistics as the tool utilized by public health professionals in the assessment of health issues in specific populations. Chapter 2 delves into the effect of the environment on human health as well as the emerging concerns for environmental justice in protecting the health hazards from government and industries on the poor, economically marginalized segments of the U.S. population. Chapter 3 addresses the use of epidemiology as a tool in public health and its primary role in assessment as well as its application in intervention designs and health policy development and health legislation. Chapter 4 presents the role of health policy and management in public health program development, implementation, and evaluation. Finally, Chapter 5 addresses the behavioral and social determinants of health, health theories, and the application of social and behavioral data in public health interventions, as well as the factors influencing health disparities.

In conclusion, because public health is an ever-changing science, we have consulted with information judged to be reliable at the time of the presentation of these materials. In spite of this, and because of the possibility of human error, the author, contributors, and publisher cannot be held responsible for any errors resulting from the use of this information. Therefore, readers are advised to consult other texts for the confirmation of the data presented herein.

We sincerely welcome suggestions, criticisms, and remarks for the improvement of this text. Contact us, and view additional public health resources, at http://www.jbpub.com.

INTRODUCTION

Public Health Science:
Principles and Practice

Larry Holmes, Jr., Doriel D. Ward, Jennifer Thompson, and John Balogun

PREVIEW

Public health emerged from the need to provide clean and safe water and protect the population from contaminated food in an attempt to reduce morbidity and mortality from infectious diseases; it remains a collective attempt by the government, public and private sectors, and individual communities to ensure that we as a society stay healthy. While there are many definitions of public health, it is simply the science and art of disease, disability and injury prevention, and health promotion at a population level.

These introductory materials address the mission, goal, substance, and core functions of public health. To achieve these core functions, the framework of public health integrates both the substance of public health, which involves disease prevention and health promotions, and the essential public health services, namely: (1) health services monitoring and identification of community health needs; (2) diagnoses and investigation of health problems and health hazards in the community; (3) informing, educating, and empowering people about health issues; (4) mobilizing community partnerships to identify and solve health problems; (5) enforcing laws and regulations that protect and ensure safety; (6) linking people with needed personal health services and ensuring the provision of health care when otherwise unavailable; (7) ensuring a competent public health and personal healthcare workforce; (8) evaluating effectiveness, accessibility, and quality of personal and population-based health services; and (9) researching new insights and innovative solutions to health problems.

The history of public health is reviewed, with the main focus on the achievement of public health during the 21st century, namely: (1) motor vehicle safety; (2) safer workplaces; (3) infectious disease control; (4) decline in coronary artery disease and stroke mortality; (5) safer and healthier food; (6) healthier mothers and babies; (7) family planning; (8) fluoridation of drinking water; (9) vaccination; and (10) recognition of tobacco as a health hazard. The challenges of public health today are also briefly mentioned: (1) aging U.S. population with the associated chronic diseases and disabilities; (2) climate changes and global warming; (3) bioterrorism and disaster preparedness; and (4) increasing health disparities.

I.   **What Is Public Health?**
   A.   Public health is the interdisciplinary science and art of disease, disability, injury prevention, and control in the human population.
      1.   Public health focuses on preventing diseases, prolonging life, and promoting physical and mental health, sanitation, personal hygiene, infection control, and organization of health services.
      2.   Public health also focuses on enhancing health in human populations through organized community efforts.
      3.   Public health is what we, as a society, do collectively to ensure that people can be healthy.
   B.   The mission of public health is to fulfill society's interest in ensuring conditions in which the people (community) can be healthy.
   C.   The goal of public health is to promote population health through shared responsibility, organized efforts, and managed care.
   D.   The core functions of public health agencies, at all levels of government, are assessment of needs and health status, policy development, and assurance of public health services.
   E.   Public health substance is disease, injury, and disability control and prevention and health promotion, achieved through organized community effort.
   F.   *Health* is defined by the World Health Organization (WHO) as the state of physical, mental, and social well-being, not the mere absence of a disease.
   G.   *Health care* is the prevention, treatment, and management of illness and the preservation of mental and physical well-being through the services offered by the medical, nursing, and allied health professions.
      1.   According to the WHO, health care embraces all the goods and services designed to promote health, including "preven-

tive, curative, and palliative interventions, whether directed to individuals or to populations."

II. **Public Health versus Medicine**
   A. Public health is concerned with the community or population, including animal populations (veterinary public health).
   B. Medicine is concerned with individual patients.
   C. Public health focuses on preventing illness, disabilities, and injuries.
   D. Medicine focuses on the treatment of individual patients.

III. **Public Health Approach to Disease and Disability and Injury Prevention**

Table 1   The Stages in Public Health Initiative in Disease, Disabilities, and Injuries Prevention at the Population Level

Stages	Description
Health problem ascertainment	Clear and unambiguous definition of the health problem
Risk/protective factors identification	Postulated and researched risk factors
Intervention development	Intervention design and pilot
Intervention implementation	Intervention conduct
Program monitoring and evaluation	Data collection, analysis, and interpretation and results dissemination

IV. **Core Functions of Public Health and Essential Public Health Services**
   A. *Core functions of public health*

Table 2   The Core Functions of Public Health

Core Function	Description
Assessment	Systematic collection
	Assembling data (processing)
	Data analyses
	Dissemination of information on the health of the community, including health status statistics, community health needs, and epidemiologic and other studies of health problems

Table 2	The Core Functions of Public Health *(continued)*
Core Function	**Description**
Policy development	The process by which society: ■ Makes decisions about problems ■ Chooses goals and the proper means to reach them ■ Handles conflicting views about what should be done ■ Allocates resources
Assurance	High-quality services, including personal health services, needed for the protection of public health are available and accessible to all persons ■ Proper allocation of state, federal, and local resources for public health ■ Availability of information on how to obtain and comply with health services requirements

B. *Essential public health services*
  1. Monitoring and identifying community health needs.
  2. Diagnosing and investigating health problems and health hazards in the community.
  3. Informing, educating, and empowering people about health issues.
  4. Mobilizing community partnerships to identify and solve health problems.
  5. Enforcing laws and regulations that protect and ensure safety.
  6. Linking people with needed personal health services and ensuring the provision of health care when otherwise unavailable.
  7. Ensuring a competent public health and personal health care workforce.
  8. Evaluating effectiveness, accessibility, and quality of personal and population-based health services.
  9. Researching new insights and innovative solutions to health problems.

V. **Origin of Public Health**
  A. *Early history*
    1. Diversion of human waste to protect public health (Ancient Rome).

2. Variolation (subcutaneous inoculation of attenuated pustule material in patients) following smallpox epidemic around 1000 B.C. (China).

3. Removing dead bodies to prevent bacterial infection during the Black Death in Europe (14th century).

4. Quarantine to mitigate infectious diseases (Medieval Europe).

5. Vaccination to treat smallpox by Edward Jenner (1820s).

6. Development of the miasma theory of disease after cholera pandemic in Europe (1829–1851).

B. *Modern history*

1. Observation of microorganisms as the cause of most infectious diseases (Anton van Leeuwenhoek, 1680).

2. Identification of polluted well water as the source of cholera epidemic in London in 1854 (John Snow). This indicated a transition from the miasma theory of disease to the germ theory and was the foundation of the science of epidemiology.

3. Germ theory—disease, single pathogen—defines a one-to-one relationship between a microorganism and the occurrence of disease (Robert Koch, mid- to late 1880s).

4. Artificial vaccine production and the theory that specific transmissible pathogens are responsible for disease (Louis Pasteur, mid-1800s).

5. Increase in average life span in late 20th- and early 21st-century United States due to public health achievements in vaccination programs and control of infectious diseases, motor vehicle and occupational safety, improved family planning, drinking water fluoridation, and smoking cessation programs.

6. Infant mortality lowering in the United States using preventive methods—i.e., feed, bathe, and dress babies (Sara Josephine Baker, 21st century).

7. HIV/AIDS epidemic (1980s) and global response to HIV/AIDS epidemic.

8. Population-level risk factors—health disparities, inequality, poverty, and education (1980s).

9. Increase in obesity and type II diabetes (United States, 1990–2000s).

10. Emerging infectious diseases such as severe acute respiratory syndrome in 2002.

11. New public health challenges to address health inequalities by addressing social determinants of health, thus narrowing and eliminating health disparities in gender, education, race, and age.
12. Advocation of policies that promote the health of the whole population in an equitable pattern (United States, 2000s).
13. Socioeconomic and social determinants of health being highly recognized (WHO, 2003).
14. Terrorism and bioterrorism preparedness (2000s).
15. Natural disaster preparedness (Katrina in United States and Tsunami in Asia, 2000s).

Table 3 — The History of Public Health

Name	Accomplishment	Date
Romans	Diversion of human waste to protect public health	
Chinese	Variation following smallpox	1000 B.C.
South Carolina	First water protection regulation	1671
South Carolina	First Health Officer	1712
Lemuel Shattuck	Review of sanitation practices, enforcement of sanitation code, and the establishment of the Massachusetts Local Board of Health	1850
John Snow	Identification of polluted water source in cholera epidemic in London	1854
Jakob Henle, Robert Koch	Disease causation based on germ theory	1880s
Edward Jenner	Vaccination to treat smallpox	1880s
South Carolina	Identification of swamp drainage as essential in stopping malaria	1881
South Carolina	Establishment of the State Board of Health	1898
Jonas Salk	Polio vaccine development reducing the number of U.S. cases from 58,000 in 1952 to 5,000 in 1957	1955

VI. Modern Functions and Accomplishments of Public Health
   A. Health surveillance, monitoring, and analysis (epidemiology and biostatistics—assessment core function).

B. Disease outbreak investigation; epidemic and disease risk factors (epidemiology and biostatistics—assessment core function).

C. Establishing, designing, and managing health promotion and disease prevention programs (policy science, epidemiology, biostatistics, behavioral sciences—policy development and assessment core functions).

D. Enabling and empowering communities to promote health and reduce inequalities (policy and management science, health promotion, and health promotion practices—policy and assurance core functions).

E. Ensuring compliance with regulations and laws to protect and promote health (management and policy science—assurance core function).

F. Creating and sustaining federal, state, local, and private sector partnership to improve health and reduce health disparities (policy and management science—policy and assurance core functions).

G. Developing and maintaining a well-educated and well-trained multidisciplinary public health task force.

H. Providing comprehensive and current information in the training of able future leaders into the field of public health.

I. Ensuring the effective performance of Healthy People 2010 objectives in improving health, preventing diseases, and eliminating health disparities.

J. Encouraging research, development, evaluation, and innovation.

K. Increasing quality assurance in public health functions.

Table 4   21st-Century Public Health Achievements in the United States

- Vaccination
- Motor vehicle safety
- Safer workplaces
- Control of infectious diseases—infant mortality reduction
- Decline in coronary health disease and stroke deaths—reduction in cigarette smoking

Table 4 21st-Century Public Health Achievements in the United States *(continued)*
■ Safer and healthier food—FDA enforcement of related federal public health laws
■ Healthier mothers and babies—improvement in maternal and child health services
■ Family planning
■ Fluoridation of drinking water
■ Recognition of tobacco as a hazard
Source: Centers for Disease Control and Prevention, http://www.cdc.gov/tobacco/mm4812.pdf

VII. Core Areas and Disciplines of Public Health

A. *Basic sciences of public health*

Table 5 Basic Sciences of Public Health: Disciplines and their Basic Components/Features	
Discipline	**Characteristics/Features**
Epidemiology: science of disease, injuries, and disabilities; distribution, determinants, and prevention in the human and related animal populations	Assessment of disease, disabilities, and injuries
	Disease distribution in human and related animal populations
	■ Persons/animals
	■ Place
	■ Time
	Measures of disease frequency
	Appropriate study designs to answer the research question(s)
	Measures disease risk (relative risk, odds ratio, prevalence odds ratio, risk ratio, hazards ratio)
	Determines disease causation (Hill and Doll's criteria, meta-analysis, factual inference)
	Determines study validity through critique and other measures
	Evidence-based risk and protective factors identification

Table 5 Basic Sciences of Public Health: Disciplines and their Basic Components/Features *(continued)*	
Discipline	**Characteristics/Features**
Biostatistics: science of inferences on random sample	Quantification of disease, disabilities, and injuries
	Sampling techniques and appropriate sample (decision on how many will be in the study)
	▪ Response rate and attrition
	▪ Power estimation
	Probability of performance/diagnostic test
	▪ Sensitivity, specificity, predictive value
	Design and analysis techniques for observational and clinical trial studies
	Hypotheses testing (parametric and nonparametric)
	Role of statistics in epidemiologic/public health research
	Inferential statistics and studies recommendation

B. *Applied sciences of public health*

Table 6 Applied Sciences of Public Health: Disciplines and their Basic Components/Features	
Discipline	**Characteristics/Features**
Behavioral and social sciences: multidisciplinary science of human actions and reactions	Health theories, models, and beliefs
	Behavioral risk and protective factors in disease
	Social determinants of diseases and racial disparities in screening, diagnosis, treatment, and prognosis
	Behavioral interventions (community-based intervention trials, education intervention, behavior modeling, and motivation to change behavior)
	Health promotions and risk avoidance (HIV/AIDS, chronic diseases, obesity, cancer, infant mortality, prenatal care, etc.)

Table 6 Applied Sciences of Public Health: Disciplines and their Basic Components/Features *(continued)*	
Discipline	**Characteristics/Features**
Environmental and occupational health: science of environmental influence on health and effect of working environment on disease, disabilities, and injuries	Impact of environment on human health, occupational injury, diseases, and mortality Environmental factors in health promotion ■ Routes and effects of exposure to environmental hazards ■ Assessment of environmental risk ■ Methods of environmental modification Major sources of environmental hazards ■ Air pollution ■ Water pollution ■ Solid waste ■ Contaminated food ■ Environmental factors ■ Weaponized pathogens Nutritional environment ■ Effect of undernutrition and overnutrition ■ Effect of excessive caloric intake and inadequate physical activities on health and disease outcomes
Management and policy science: decision making on intervention goal and resources allocation	Policy development and public health Factors affecting public health Administration of public health Goals of public health

VIII. Challenges of Public Health

    A. *Global warming*

        1. Climate warming and human health with the consequences being:

            a. Emerging hyperthermia.

            b. Emerging infections.

            c. Heat stroke, especially in individuals compromised by diseases or cardiovascular disorders, and the elderly.

            d. Cutaneous malignancy.

      e. Increase in air and water pollution, resulting in infectious diseases.

      f. Asthma and pulmonary congestion.

  2. These conditions are likely to involve the socioeconomically marginalized segments of the U.S. population, mainly ethnic/racial minorities.

GLOBAL WARMING AND PUBLIC HEALTH IMPLICATIONS

- There is an association between seasonal variation and human health, including mental health.
- Extreme temperatures can result in failure in the thermoregulatory center, hypothalamus, leading to death.
- Hospital data on admission on mortality indicate increasing rate of deaths during extremely hot days especially among elderly, young children, and those with chronic diseases.
- Also, extreme temperature can lead to an increase in air and water pollution and the subsequent infectious diseases such as West Nile Virus, Cholera, and Lyme disease (pathogens affiliated with high heat as seen in summer).
- The physical effect of climate change is the alteration in the air temperature, thus increasing the concentration of ozone at ground level.
- Exposure to ozone especially by those with already compromised cardio-respiratory function may result in chest pain and pulmonary congestion.

B. *Aging America*

  1. Aging population is predisposed to chronic disabilities and chronic disease and malignancies.

  2. Public health is charged with implementing programs to address lifestyle variables and decrease chronic disabilities and illnesses and promote successful aging and disease-free longevity.

C. *Obesity and overweight*

  1. More than 66% of the U.S. population is overweight or obese; the consequences of obesity and overweight are:

      a. Type II diabetes.

      b. Cardiovascular diseases.

      c. Some cancers.

d.   Preterm and low birth weights, congenital anomalies, and infant mortality.

e.   Maternal morbidity (gestational diabetes, pre-eclampsia).

2.   Public health is charged with preventing obesity by behavioral intervention to address excessive caloric intake and enhance regular and moderate exercise.

PUBLIC HEALTH CHALLENGES IN THE MILLENIUM

EMERGING AND RESISTANT PATHOGEN—Public health is threatened with the emerging infections and the antibiotic resistance associated with the changes in the envelop proteins of these pathogens, as they continue to mutate.

OBESITY EPIDEMIC—The epidemic of obesity and overweight presents a great challenge to public health and requires research and behavioral interventions in addressing its behavioral and lifestyle components.

- Realistically, the life expectancy gained by this nation in the areas of heart diseases and stroke as a result of tobacco cessation and lifestyle modification in this direction will be lost to obesity epidemic.
- Public health agencies need to act now in reducing the epidemic of obesity and overweight.

AGING AMERICA—Aging is not a pathologic process but is associated with a decline in biologic systems.

- To address successful aging, public health needs to prevent chronic diseases and chronic disabilities in the first place and compress morbidity.
- To achieve successful aging or disease-free longevity is a challenge to public health in any society with an increase in the aging population.

HEALTH DISPARITIES—The increasing disparities in health with racial/ethnic minorities, mainly African Americans, being disproportionately burdened, is indicative of the need for equitable provision of public health services to such vulnerable populations.

SOCIO-ECONOMIC INEQUITY—Public health is challenged with confronting health with politics and allocating resources to those who can not afford health in our society.

GLOBAL WARMING—Excessive alteration in ambient temperature is associated with increased acute and chronic diseases, hospitalization, and mortality. The rising environmental temperature and factors associated with it need to be addressed by a responsible public health system.

D. *Terrorism*
1. Whereas public health is not designed to control or prevent terrorism, public health is charged with the responsibility of responding to such attacks by coordinating services needed to reduce casualties and respond to the attack, thus preventing further damages to human health and loss of human lives.

E. *Disaster preparedness*
1. Disasters that public health cannot control, and the response to the aftermath of such disasters, remain the responsibilities of public health.
2. A prompt response to disasters such as Katrina in New Orleans and the tsunami in Asia requires a well-coordinated disaster preparedness effort from the public health services.

F. *Health disparities elimination*
1. Healthy People 2010 focuses on health disparities elimination.
2. Public health is charged with the responsibility of providing equitable preventive services to all sectors of the population, especially the socioeconomically marginalized, children, women, elderly, and racial and ethnic minorities.
3. Realistically, the future of the U.S. population's health depends on the collective and shared effort of public health agencies to develop and enforce policies that will ensure the provision of health services to all at a population level, regardless of the ability to afford such services (e.g., immunization as primary prevention of vaccine-preventable diseases).

G. *Community participatory research, translational research, and environmental justice*
1. *Community participatory research* advocates the involvement of the community in research planning, conduct, and evaluation. The community provides data for public health assessment of needs, risks, benefits, and resources. Public health programs' development, implementation, and evaluation must involve the community. Communities must provide informed consent for research to be conducted. This is, in part, the notion behind community participatory research.
   a. Further, public health research findings must be shared with the community. Public health is faced with applying

community participatory research in addressing interventions designed to benefit the community.

2. *Translational research* is at the center of the benefits of research at the community level. The ultimate purpose of research is to improve the health status of the community by applying what is known at the intervention trial to the routine practice at the community level. The barriers to this translation had recently been the focus of the National Institutes of Health.

   a. Public health is challenged with designing measures that will facilitate the application of research findings in public health to the community on routine use, away from the trial or controlled environment that does not represent the real-world situation.

3. *Environmental justice* advocates the role of the popular movement, the poor in the improvement of public health, and the recognition of the contribution of this movement to the achievement of public health in this nation. Economically marginalized segments of our population are disproportionately burdened by the adverse effect of toxic environment on health. The poor physical environment tends to be identified with toxic waste deposition by the government and the industry.

   a. Environmental justice represents the movement to reduce the burden of environmental health on the vulnerable and poor segment of our population.

4. Public health is challenged with including those who live in these environmentally "unsafe" environments in the decision to improve their health, because the will or desire (motivation) to remain healthy is essential in any effort to control disease and improve health.

REFERENCES

Centers for Disease Control and Prevention. Achievements in public health, 1900–1999: Changes in the public health system. *MMWR.* 1998;48(50):1141–1147.

Centers for Disease Control and Prevention. Control of infectious diseases. *MMWR.* 1999;48:621–629.

Centers for Disease Control and Prevention. Decline in deaths from heart disease and stroke—United States, 1900–1999. *MMWR.* 1999;48:649–656.

Centers for Disease Control and Prevention. *Eliminating Racial & Ethnic Health Disparities.* http://www.cdc.gov/omhd. Accessed November 15, 2007.

Centers for Disease Control and Prevention. Family planning. *MMWR.* 1999;48: 1073–1080.

Centers for Disease Control and Prevention. Fluoridation of drinking water to prevent dental caries. *MMWR.* 1999;48:933–940.

Centers for Disease Control and Prevention. Healthier mothers and babies. *MMWR.* 1999;48:849–857.

Centers for Disease Control and Prevention. Impact of vaccines universally recommended for children—United States, 1990–1998. *MMWR.* 1999;48:243–248.

Centers for Disease Control and Prevention. Improvements in workplace safety—United States, 1900–1999. *MMWR.* 1999;48:461–469.

Centers for Disease Control and Prevention. Motor-vehicle safety: A 20th century public health achievement. *MMWR.* 1999;48:369–374.

Centers for Disease Control and Prevention. Safer and healthier foods. *MMWR.* 1999;48:905–913.

Centers for Disease Control and Prevention. Ten great public health achievements in the United States, 1900–1999. *MMWR.* 1999;48:241–243.

Centers for Disease Control and Prevention. Tobacco use—United States, 1900–1999. *MMWR.* 1999;48:986–993.

Committee on Assuring the Health of the Public in the 21st Century. *The Future of the Public's Health in the 21st Century.* Washington, DC: National Academy Press; 2002.

Flies JL. *Statistical Methods for Rates and Proportions.* 2nd ed. New York: John Wiley & Sons; 1981.

Glik DC. *Bioterrorism Preparedness: Workforce, Organizational, Resources, and Risk Communication Issues.* Presented at American Public Health Association, 132nd Annual Meeting, November 6–10, 2004, Washington, DC.

Institute of Medicine. *Healthy Communities.* Washington, DC: National Academy Press; 1996.

Institute of Medicine. *The Future of Public Health.* Washington, DC: National Academy Press; 1988.

Motulsky H. *Intuitive Biostatistics.* New York: Oxford University Press; 1995.

Ory MG. *Emerging Issues in Geriatric Care: Aging and Public Health Perspectives.* Presented at American Public Health Association, 132nd Annual Meeting, November 6–10, 2004, Washington, DC.

Riscia PM. *Prevention of Overweight and Obesity: Focus on Children and Adolescents.* Presented at American Public Health Association, 132nd Annual Meeting, November 6–10, 2004, Washington, DC.

Roemer MI. Preparing public health leaders for the 1990s. *Public Health Rep.* 1988;103:443–451.

Schneider M. *Introduction to Public Health.* 2nd ed. Sudbury, MA: Jones and Bartlett; 2006.

Scutchfield DF, Keck W. *Principles of Public Health Practice.* New York: Delmar Series in Health Services; 2002.

Senior PA, Bhopal R. Ethnicity as a variable in epidemiological research. *BMJ*. 1994; 309:327–330.

U.S. Global Change Research Program. *A Report of the National Assessment Synthesis Team, Climate Change Impacts on the United States—The Potential Consequences of Climate Variability and Change*. http://www.usgcrp.gov/usgcrp/naac. Accessed November 12, 2007.

Winkelstein W, French FE. The training of epidemiologists in schools of public health in the United States: A historical note. *Int J Epidemiol*. 1973;2:415–416.

Principles and Methods of Biostatistics

Larry Holmes, Jr.

BIOSTATISTICS CORE COMPETENCIES LEARNING OBJECTIVES

Biostatistics is the development and application of statistical reasoning and methods in addressing, analyzing, and solving problems in public health; health care; and biomedical, clinical, and population-based research.

PHCC.1.1.	Describe the roles biostatistics serves in the discipline of public health.
PHCC.1.2.	Distinguish among the different measurement scales and the implications for selection of statistical methods to be used based on these distinctions.
PHCC.1.3.	Apply descriptive techniques commonly used to summarize public health data.
PHCC.1.4.	Describe basic concepts of probability, random variation, and commonly used statistical probability distributions.
PHCC.1.5.	Apply common statistical methods for inference.
PHCC.1.6.	Describe preferred methodological alternatives to commonly used statistical methods when assumptions are not met.
PHCC.1.7.	Apply descriptive and inferential methodologies according to the type of study design for answering a particular research question.
PHCC.1.8.	Interpret results of statistical analyses found in public health studies.

PHCC.1.9.	Develop written and oral presentations based on statistical analyses for both public health professionals and educated lay audiences.
PHCC.1.10.	Apply basic information techniques with vital statistics and public health records in the description of public health characteristics and in public health research and evaluation.

PREVIEW

Biostatistics is a tool for the epidemiologic assessment and monitoring of health status, needs, and risk factors in order for public health to fulfill its substance of disease control and health promotions. As a basic science of public health, *biostatistics* has been described as the development and application of statistical reasoning and methods in addressing, analyzing, and solving problems in public health [**PHCC1.1**]; health care; and biomedical, clinical, and population-based research. Both descriptive and inferential statistics are essential components of applied statistics in public health research.

This chapter presents the basic notion of statistics and the role of statistics in health, biological, and medical sciences. Distinction is made between descriptive statistics (measures and central tendencies and dispersions) and inferential statistics (hypothesis testing and conclusion from the sample). Vignettes are utilized to illustrate the application of the classic statistical notions to real-world situation. Several test statistics are presented with their assumptions and rationale in testing various hypotheses and addressing relevant research questions. The statistical techniques or methods are reviewed in detail (correlation analysis, linear regression, logistic regression, and Cox proportional hazards model). Logistic regression analysis is reviewed with examples, given its widespread use in public health. The critique of literature is presented with the intent to allow readers to grasp the practical importance of biostatistics in the appraisal of scientific literature. Finally, reference is made to the section of the core competencies covered in the text, such as PHCC.1.2, that presents the scales of measurement of variables and their implication in the selection of test statistics.

I. **Statistics and Biostatistics**
    A. *Biostatistics/biometry:* statistics applied to biological sciences and health-related events. This involves:
        1. Making sense of health-related data. [PHCC.1.1]
        2. Making inference about a population of interest based on information obtained from a sample of measurements from that population remains the objective of applied statistics such as biostatistics.
    B. *Statistics:* concerned with data (numbers that contain information) collection, management (organization), analysis, and interpretation.
        1. Statistics studies a sample of the population; thus, drawing inferences about a population is a major role of statistics in research.
        2. Statistics is used to objectify the conclusions made in observational and experimental studies in public health. [PHCC.1.1]
    C. Statistical methods are used in public health to (1) measure and explain overall variation, (2) differentiate between random and meaningful variation, and (3) facilitate the interpretation of data needed for risk factors understanding and intervention implementation. [PHCC.1.1]
    D. Biostatistics is the branch of applied statistics that investigates and evaluates the nature of information gathered on biological, clinical, and health issues or conditions.
        1. The role of biostatistics in research commences from design of study through implementation and the manuscript preparation for results dissemination. [PHCC.1.1]

II. **Population Characteristics**
    A. Statistics is about sampling, and sampling is used to estimate or approximate the "real" or "true" characteristics of the population under investigation or study.
    B. *Sample* refers to cases, subjects, or study participants (smaller group or subset of population) who are selected from the larger group (population) to investigate the association between exposure and disease (e.g., to understand the association in the population, also termed *source population* in this illustration).
        1. *Vignette:* Consider a study to examine the association between blood pressure and oral contraceptives. If the investigator

selects 200 undergraduate female students in a university with 5,000 female students, the sample represents the 200 female students. The result of the study will be used to draw inference on the entire population (5,000 female students).

C. *Scales used to measure population characteristics:* refers to a variable (entity that varies) or sets of values that can be described and analyzed statistically. [PHCC.1.2]

1. *Continuous* (can assume an infinite number of values) refers to a measure that uses an infinite number of values [e.g., weight, systolic blood pressure (millimeters), urine drug concentration, hematocrit (millimeters), height (centimeters), body mass index (BMI) (kg/m^2), etc.].

2. *Discrete* (finite number of intervals) refers to only a few possible values, and measured in categories or classes [e.g., number of cigars/day, sex (male/female), race, marital status, skin color].

3. *Ordinal* (ordered categories) refers to categorical measures with natural order (e.g., educational status, socioeconomic status, pain level, comorbidity index, and disease severity).

4. *Dichotomous* refers to categorical measurements that contain only two classes (e.g., presence or absence of a disease). Hypertension may be coded as (presence = 1) and (absence = 0).

BOX 1-1   TYPES OF VARIABLES

- Outcome—provided the response to another variable that is said to be a predictor. Also termed response
- Explanatory—determines the changes in the response variable. Otherwise termed independent or predictor variable

---

D. *Estimates* are the values of sample characteristics, so termed because they proximate the value in the larger population. [PHCC.1.2]

E. *Continuous* characteristics in a population are described with the *mean* and *standard deviation* (measure of how much individual values in the population vary from the mean)—appropriate descriptive statistics for continuous variables. [PHCC.1.2]

F. *Discrete* or categorical characteristics from a population are described with proportion or percentage and rate (special proportion with time as a denominator). [PHCC.1.2]

G. *Ordinal* characteristics in a population are described by using median (population midpoint of ordered data) or mode (most frequent value). [PHCC.1.2]

H. *Probability model* is used to infer the characteristics of the population from the sample inferential statistics, which attempts to answer the question as to whether the observed difference is a result of "chance."

I. *Accuracy* with respect to the sample estimate refers to how close the estimate is to the true value in the population from which the sample was obtained; it is the ability of measurement to be correct on average.

J. *Bias* is a systematic or differential error in an estimate, with the sources of bias including:

1. *Selection bias,* occurring when the subjects selected for study are not representative of the source population, limiting generalization of the result.[1]

2. *Misclassification/information bias,* which may result from:

   a. Defect or inaccuracy in the measuring device.

   b. Inaccuracy in the observation or recording of the measurements.[2]

K. *Precision* (degree of "chance" differential or random error), also termed *reproducibility, consistency, replicability,* or *reliability,* refers to the variability in the estimate. A measurement could be precise and not accurate, accurate and not precise, precise and accurate, or inaccurate and imprecise. Study precision is affected by random error, and could result from (1) observer variability, (2) subject variability, (3) instrument variability, or (4) instability of the attribute being measured. [PHCC.1.4]

L. *Standard deviation* (SD) refers to the ability of a measurement to give the same results or very similar results with repeated measurements of the same thing. For example, the greater the SD, the less precise an estimate the mean will be from the true population mean (μ). [PHCC.1.4]

M. *Reliability studies* are designed to quantify the reproducibility of the same variable (e.g., daily dietary intake of a particular food), measured more than once. Kappa, which is a measure of agreement "beyond chance," is used as a measure of reproducibility between repeated assessments of the same variable. The chi-square test of association between the two survey responses, although performable, will not give a quantitative measure of the reproducibility between the responses at the two surveys. Using kappa statistics (κ) is the appropriate test to measure reproducibility: $P_o - P_e / 1 - P_e$, where P_o is the observed probability of the concordance between two surveys, and P_e is the expected probability of concordance between the two surveys. Kappa, $\kappa > 0.75$ (75%) indicates excellent reproducibility, 0.4 (40%) $\leq \kappa \leq 0.75$ (75%) indicates good reproducibility, while $0 \leq \kappa < 0.4$ (40%) denotes marginal/poor reproducibility. In addition, $+1.0$ is indicative of a perfect agreement, while 0.0 indicates complete independence between the two surveys. Specificity and sensitivity would be more appropriate indices of reliability or reproducibility if the investigators were interested in the concordance between responses on two different variables, where one of the variables is considered to be the cold standard.[3]

N. The degree of precision or random error is measured by the size of its confidence interval (CI), that is, the range of values for which one is fairly confident/certain that the true value from the population lies. [PHCC.1.4]

O. CI can be computed using the standard error (SE), which is the function of variability in the sample.

1. SE is measured by SD and the sample size (n). Mathematically, $SE = SD / \sqrt{n}$, where n is the sample size.[4,5]

BOX 1-2   STANDARD NORMAL DISTRIBUTION

- Standard normal distribution n (0,1)
- Mean = 0 and Standard Deviation (SD) = 1
- Z (standardized variable) $= x - \mu / \sigma$
- Where μ is the mean, and σ is the SD

III. Descriptive Statistics

A. Making sense of data in public health research involves four basic steps: (1) data collection, (2) data summary, (3) data analysis, and (4) data interpretation/result presentation. [PHCC.1.1]

B. Summarizing data, organizing data, graphing, and describing numeric information are the functions of descriptive statistics.

C. Descriptive statistics is concerned with measures of central tendencies and measures of dispersion, as well as their graphic presentation.

1. A *parameter* is a measurement of a population that characterizes one of its features. An example of a parameter is the mode. The mode is the value in the population that occurs most frequently. Other examples of parameters are a population's mean (or average) and its variance.[5]

2. Parameter has been referred to as certain summary constant that describes the population or universe.[6]

3. Descriptive statistics refers to *parameters* [population value of a characteristic of a *distribution* (values of characteristics or variable along with the frequency of their occurrence)] used to describe the attributes of a set of data such as mean, SD, proportion, and rate. [PHCC.1.4]

Table 1-1	Scales of Measurement/Types of Variables*	
Type of Data	**Description and Example**	**Sample Estimate Summary and Presentation**
Nominal (qualitative)	Dichotomous, binary, categorical	Proportion, percentage displayed with bar chart, contingency table
Ordinal	Nominal scale with natural order; e.g., stage of tumors	Proportion and percentage, median, mode; displayed with bar chart, contingency table
Numerical (quantitative)	Continuous or interval and discrete	Mean and standard deviation, median and mode; displayed with stem and leaf plot, histograms, box plots, frequency polygons, and percentage polygons

*The scale of measurement influences the summary and the display of information. Variable refers to any information that can vary.

D. *Vignette:* Consider a chemoprevention study to assess the protective effect of selenium in prostate cancer. To test this hypothesis, investigators collected data from 500 treatments and 500 controls.

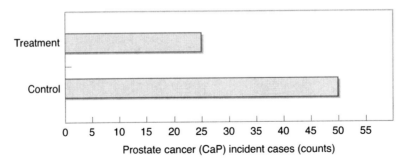

Figure 1-1   Incidence of Prostate Cancer Among Healthy U.S. Male Adults in Selenium Chemoprevention Trial (Hypothetical Study)

What should be the initial approach toward understanding these data at the end of the intervention?

E.   *Solution:* Prior to analysis of these data, a bar graph could be used to show those in the control who developed prostate cancer relative to the treatment group at the end of the follow-up.

F.   *Measures of central tendency* [PHCC.1.3]

1.   The mean, median, and mode are the commonly used measures of location or central tendency.

2.   Whereas the *mean* (arithmetic mean) is the most commonly used measure of location, it is sensitive to extreme value (outliers) or skewed distribution, which makes it an inappropriate measure of central location in these types of samples.

3.   Mathematically, the mean is calculated by summing all the observations and dividing by the number of observations.

4.   Mean = $\Sigma X / n$, where Σ is the summation, X is the observation, and n is the number of observations.

   a.   *Vignette:* Consider systolic blood pressure (SBP) of 10 women diagnosed with angina pectoris in a cardiovascular clinic ($x_1 = 102$, $x_2 = 144$, $x_3 = 110$, $x_4 = 138$, $x_5 = 130$, $x_6 = 120$, $x_7 = 140$, $x_8 = 100$, $x_9 = 60$, $x_{10} = 106$). What is the mean SBP in this sample?

   b.   *Solution:* Mean (arithmetic) = Sum of the SBP / Number of SBP (subjects). Substituting: $(x_1 + x_2 + x_3 \ldots x_{10}) / n \rightarrow 115$.

5.   *Median* is the middle value in ordered or arranged data.

   a.   It is an appropriate measure of central location when the data have outliers (skewed data).

      b. *Skewed distribution* refers to outlying observations occurring in only one direction; thus, there are either a few small values or a few large values.

      c. *Positive skewness* occurs if the outlying values are large; thus, the distribution is skewed to the right.

      d. *Negative skewness* occurs if the outlying values are small; thus, the distribution is skewed to the left.

6. *Mode* is the item with the highest frequency, or the value most frequently attained in a sample or population.

      a. Both the mode and median are not influenced by extremely high or low values or observations; thus, they are useful in describing continuous variables/scale data whose values are not "normally" distributed. [PHCC.1.3]

Table 1-2 Uses of Measures of Location/Central Tendency*	
Measures of Location	**Statistical Utility**
Mean	Numerical data
	Symmetric (nonskewed) data (distribution)
	Observations measured on a log scale (geometric mean)
Median	Ordinal data
	Numerical data with skewed distribution
Mode	Binomial distribution
*Suggestive of which measure of central tendency is best with a given set of data.	

G. *Measures of dispersion* [PHCC.1.3]

1. Measures of dispersion/spread are variance and standard deviation. Other measures of dispersion/variation are range, coefficient of variation, percentile rank, and interquartile range.

2. Range is the difference between the largest and the smallest observations.

      a. *Vignette:* Consider the lowest mean arterial blood pressure (mmHg) of cocaine-dependent patients in a drug rehabilitation clinic to be 108 and the highest to be 131. What is the range?

      b. *Solution:* The range is computed by subtracting the maximum from the minimum value. Substituting: $131 - 108 \rightarrow 23$ mmHg.

3. *Coefficient of variation (CV)* is a useful measure of relative variation or spread in data.
4. CV is mathematically given by $SD/X \times 100 \to SD/X(100)$, where *SD* is the standard deviation and *X* is the mean. This is a measure of relative variation, or the variation that is relative to the size of the mean.
5. CV is useful in laboratory testing and quality control procedures.
6. *Percentile* is the percentage of a distribution that is equal to or below a particular number.
    a. It is used to compare individual value such as height with the norm (e.g., a growth chart).
7. *Interquartile range* is the measure of variation that utilizes percentiles (e.g., the first and third quartiles are the 25th and 75th percentiles, respectively).
8. *Variance (square of SD)* is the standard dispersion of each observation from the group mean.
    a. Sum of squares / Sample size $- 1(n - 1)$, where $n - 1$ is the degree of freedom.
    b. $S^2 = \Sigma(X - M)^2 / n - 1$, where *M* is the mean of the sample, and S^2 is the biased estimate of $\sigma^2 = \Sigma(X - \mu)^2 / n$, where σ^2 is the variance in the population.[5] But because samples are used to estimate the parameters, S^2 is the most commonly used variance.
9. Because the computation of variance involves the square of the dispersion of the observation from the mean, it does not provide a true measure of the average distance of each observation from the group mean.
10. *Standard deviation (SD) is the measure of variability, implying the differences among subjects or cases.* This is the square root of the variance $\to \sqrt{\text{population variance}}$. The larger the SD, the greater the variability (spread or dispersion).[7] Assuming a normal distribution, an estimated 34% of the subjects or cases will lie within 1 SD unit of the mean. Therefore, if $X = 25.0$ and $SD = 5.0$, then 68% of the subjects lie within ± 5 points of the mean (1 SD = 68% lies between 20.0 and 30.0).
11. *Mathematically:* $\sigma = \sqrt{\Sigma(X - \mu)^2 / n}$

12. Square root of the average of the squared deviations of the observations from their mean is a more useful measure of dispersion for hypothesis testing.

Table 1-3   Steps to Calculate Variance and SD

- Calculate the mean, X.
- Prepare a table that subtracts the mean from each observed value $(X - M)$.
- Square each of the differences (different column) $(X - M)^2$.
- Add this column (sum of the squared dispersion from the mean) $\Sigma(X - M)^2$.
- Divide by $n - 1$ where n is the number of items in the sample (number of observations).
- This is the *variance*: $(S^2) \rightarrow (X - M)^2 / n - 1$.
- To get the *standard deviation*, obtain the square root of the variance: $\sqrt{(X - M)^2 / n - 1}$.

---

    a. Standard error simply stated as standard error of the mean is given by: $\sigma_m = \sigma / \sqrt{N}$, where σ_m is the SD of the sampling distribution of the mean, σ is the SD of the original distribution, and N is the sample size (not assuming normal distribution).

    b. *Standard error differs from standard deviation*: (1) SE is the SD of a population of sample means, rather than of the individual observations; (2) refers to variability of the means, rather than variability of individual observations; and (3) provides an idea of how variable a single estimate of the mean is likely to be. [PHCC.1.4]

Table 1-4   Uses of Measures of Dispersion

Measures of Dispersion	Statistical Utility
Standard deviation (SD)	Continuous data
	Mean
	Numerical data without skewness (symmetric numeric data)

Table 1-4 Uses of Measures of Dispersion *(continued)*	
Measures of Dispersion	**Statistical Utility**
Percentile and interquartile range	With median (ordinal or skewed data)
	With mean (to compare individual observations with sets of numbers)
Interquartile range	To describe the central 50% of a distribution regardless of its shape
Range	With numerical data to stress extreme values
Coefficient of variation	To compare numerical distributions measured on different scales

IV. Types of Distribution

Table 1-5 Types of Distribution	
Types of Distribution	**Description and Example(s)**
Normal (Gaussian)	Displayed as bell curve
	Data cluster around the middle or mean
	Fewer observations at either extreme
Parametric (also type of analysis, e.g., ANOVA)	Distributions that can be analyzed or estimated using parameters such as the mean and standard deviation, when the scale of measure or variable is continuous (e.g., *Z*-score, *t*-test, ANOVA)
Nonparametric (also type of analysis, e.g., chi-square)	Data that cannot be characterized by parameters such as mean and standard deviation
	Data that use nonparametric method such as chi-square

V. Performance and Screening Test [PHCC.1.4, 1.5]

   A. Screening is an effort to detect disease that is not readily apparent or risk factors for a disease in an at-risk segment of the population. This test can result in four possible outcomes or results (1) true positive—positive test with the presence of disease,

(2) false positive—positive test in the absence of disease, (3) false negative—positive test in the absence of disease, and (4) true negative—negative test in the absence of disease.

B. Diagnostic test, results, and implications of screening depend on both the prevalence of the disease and test performance.

C. Rare diseases are associated with relatively frequent false-positives relative to true-negatives.

D. Common diseases are associated with relatively frequent false-negatives relative to true-negatives.

E. Screening test is generally inappropriate when disease is either exceedingly rare or extremely common.

F. Measures of the diagnostic value of a test are its *sensitivity* and *specificity.* These parameters have important implications for screening and clinical guidelines.[8]

Table 1-6   2 × 2 Table Comparing Test Results and Disease Status

Test Result	Disease Status		
	Diseased	Nondiseased	Total
Positive	a (diseased and positive)	b (disease-free and positive)	a + b (all positive)
Negative	c (diseased and negative)	d (disease-free and negative)	c + d (all negative)
Total	a + c (all diseased)	b + d (all nondiseased)	a + b + c + d

G. *Sensitivity* refers to the ability of a test to detect a disease when it is present.
   1. Measures the proportion of those with disease who are correctly classified as diseased by the test.
   2. Sensitivity = $a / a + c$ [Subjects with true-positive test results / (Subjects with true-positive results + Subjects with false-negative test result)].
   3. A test that is not sensitive is likely to generate a false-negative result (c). False-negative error rate, $Pr(T-|D+) = c / (a + c)$, otherwise termed beta error rate or type II error.
   4. Sensitivity $[a / (a + c)]$ + False-negative error rate (FN rate), $[c / (a + c)] = 1.0$ (100%).

> **BOX 1-3   RELATIONSHIP BETWEEN DISEASE PREVALENCE, SENSITIVITY, SPECIFICITY, & PREDICTIVE VALUE**
>
> - There is a relationship between disease prevalence, sensitivity, specificity, and predictive values.
> - The prevalence simply means the probability of the condition before performing the test (i.e., pretest probability).
> - The predictive values refer to the probability of the disease being present or absent after obtaining the results of the test.
> - Using the 2 × 2 table, positive predictive value (PPV) is the proportion of those with a positive test who have the disease ($a / (a + b)$) while the negative predictive value (NPV) is the proportion of those with a negative test who do not have the disease ($d / (c + d)$).
> - The predictive values will vary with the prevalence of the disease or condition being tested for.
> - Therefore the probability of the diseases before (prevalence) and the probability of disease after (predictive value) will be interrelated, with the differences in predictive values driven by the differences in the prevalence of the disease.

   H. *Specificity* refers to the ability of test to indicate nondisease (disease-free) when no disease is present.
1. Measures the proportion of those without disease who are correctly classified as disease-free by the test.
2. Specificity $= d / (b + d)$ [Subjects with true-negative test results / (Subjects with true-negative result + Subjects with false-positive)].
3. A test that is not specific is likely to generate false-positive results (b). False-positive error rate, $Pr(T+ |D-) = b / b + d$(FP rate).
4. Specificity $(d / b + d) +$ FP rate $b / (b + d) = 1.0 (100\%)$.

   I. *Predictive values* refer to (1) the probability of having the disease being tested for if the test result is positive and (2) the probability of not having the disease being tested for if the result is negative.[9]

   J. There are two types of predictive values used in diagnostic/screening tests:
1. *Positive predictive value (PPV):* the probability of a test being positive given that the disease is present.
2. Mathematically: PD+ or PPV $= a / \{a + [(pT+ |D-)pD-)]\} = a / \{a + b\}$.

K. PD+ = True-positives / {True-positives + False-positives}. Using Bayes's theorem, PPV is the probability that an individual with a positive test result truly has disease, which is the proportion of all positives (true and false) that are true-positives.

L. PPV is thus the probability that a positive test result truly indicates the presence of disease.

BOX 1-4   POSITIVE PREDICTIVE VALUE (PPV/PV+)

- A measure of diagnostic test.
- The positive predictive value (PPV) answers the question, if the patients test result is positive, what is the probability that he or she has the disease?
- For example, if in a 2 × 2 contingency table assessing MRI and brain attack, A = 112 (true positive) and B = 20 (false positive).
- PPV indicates the proportion of the subjects who had positive MRI, and had brain attack.
- Using the formula: PPV = A / (A + B), substituting, 112 / (112 + 20) = 0.85 (85%).

M. *Sensitivity:* the probability of a positive test in those with the disease is the sensitivity ($a / a = c$).

N. *Prevalence:* the probability of the disease is the *prevalence* of the disease ($(a + c) / (a + b + c + d)$).

O. Using Bayesian theorem: PD+ = (Sensitivity × Prevalence) / {[Sensitivity × Prevalence] + [(1 − Specificity)(1 − Prevalence)]}.

P. *Negative predictive value (NPV),* or PD−, is the probability of disease absence following a negative test result.
    1. NPV = True-negatives / {True negatives + False-negatives} → $d / (d + b)$.

Q. *Using Bayesian theorem:* PD− = [Specificity × (1 − Prevalence)] / {[Specificity × (1 − Prevalence)] + [Prevalence × (1 − Sensitivity)]}.

R. *Likelihood ratios*
    1. *Likelihood ratio positive (LR+)* refers to the ratio of the sensitivity of a test to the false-positive error rate of the test.
        a. *Mathematically:* LR+ = [$a / (a + c)$] / [$b / (b + d)$].
        b. LR+ = Sensitivity / (1 − Specificity).

2. *Likelihood ratio negative (LR−)* refers to the ratio of false-negative error rate to the specificity of the test.
   a. *Mathematically:* LR− = {c / (a + c)} / {d / (b + d)}.
   b. LR− = (1 − Sensitivity) / Specificity.

S. Ratio of LR+ to LR− refers to the measure of separation between the positive and negative test.

T. Mathematically, LR+ to LR− ratio = LR+ / LR−. This is an approximation of the odds ratio. OR = *ad / bc* using 2 × 2 contingency table.
   1. *Odds ratio:* Odds of exposure in the disease / odds of exposure in the nondisease.
   2. Odds of disease (lung cancer) = Probability that lung cancer will occur (P) / Probability that it will not occur (1 − P).

U. *Vignette:* Consider 160 persons appearing in a deep vein thrombosis (DVT) clinic for lower extremities Doppler ultrasound study. If 24 out of 40 subjects with DVT tested positive for DVT, and 114 out of 120 without DVT tested negative, calculate: (1) sensitivity, (2) specificity, (3) false-positive error rate, (4) false-negative error rate, (5) positive predictive value, (6) negative predictive value, (7) likelihood ratio positive, (8) likelihood ratio negative, (9) ratio of LR+ to LR−, and (10) the prevalence of DVT.

V. Generate a 2 × 2 contingency table.

Table 1-7   2 × 2 Table for DVT and Non-DVT

Test Result	Disease Status		
	DVT	**Non-DVT**	**Total**
Positive	24	6	30
Negative	16	114	130
Total	40	120	160

W. *Computation:* (1) Sensitivity = 24 / 40 = 0.6 (60%); (2) Specificity = 0.95 (95%); (3) FP error rate = b / (b + d) = 6 / 120 = 0.05 (5%); (4) FN error rate = c / (a + c) = 16 / 40 = 0.4 (40%); (5) PPV = 24(a) / 30(a + b) = 0.8(80%); (6) NPV = 114(d) / 130(c + d) = 0.88 (88%); (7) LR+ = {a / (a + c)} = Sensitivity / {b / (b + b)}

(False-positive error rate) → 0.6 / 0.05 = 12.0; (8) LR− = False-negative error rate {(c / (a + c) / Specificity {d / (d + b)} → 0.4 / 0.95 = 0.42; (9) LR+ to LR− ratio = LR+ / LR− = 12 / 0.42 = 28.57; and (10) Prevalence of DVT = (a + c) / (a + b + c + d) → 40 / 160 = 0.25 (25%). False-positive error rate (alpha error rate or type I error rate) simply refers to an error committed by asserting that a proposition is *true*, when it is indeed *not true* (false). If a test is not *specific*, this will lead to the test falsely indicating the presence of a disease in nondisease subjects (cell B; see accompanying table). The rate at which this occurs is termed the false-positive error rate and is mathematically given by B / (B + D). False-positive error rate is related to specificity: FP rate + Specificity = 1.0(100%).

X. In summary, the prevalence simply means the probability of the condition before performing the test, meaning pretest probability. The predictive values refer to the probability of the disease being present or absent after obtaining the results of the test. Using the 2 × 2 table, PPV is the proportion of those with a positive test who have the disease [a / (a + b)], while the NPV is the proportion of those with a negative test who do not have the disease [d / (c + d)]. The predictive values will vary with the prevalence of the disease or condition being tested for. Therefore, the probability of the diseases before (prevalence) and the probability of disease after (predictive value) will be interrelated, with the differences in predictive values driven by the differences in the prevalence of the disease. Sensitivity and specificity are properties of a diagnostic test and should be consistent when the test is used in similar patients and in similar settings. Predictive values, although related to the sensitivity and specificity of the test, will vary with the prevalence of the condition or disease being tested. The difference in the sensitivity and specificity of the test is most likely as a result of the test not being administered in similar conditions (patients and settings).[10]

Y. Multiple or sequential testing refers to:
1. *Parallel testing* (ordering test together).
    a. The rationale is to increase sensitivity, but specificity is compromised.
    b. There are four possible outcomes in parallel testing: (1) T1+ T2+ (disease is present), (2) T1+ T2− (further

testing), (3) T1− T2+ (further testing), and (4) T1− T2−
(disease is absent).[11]

(1) Sensitivity (net) = (Sensitivity T1 + Sensitivity T2) −
Sensitivity T1 × Sensitivity T2.

(2) Specificity (net) = Specificity T1 × Specificity T2.

(3) Individual tested positive on either test is classified
as positive.

(4) Appropriate when false-negative is main concern.

2. *Serial testing* refers to using two tests in series, with test 2 performed only on those individuals who are positive on test 1.[11]

a. There are four possible outcomes in parallel testing:

(1) T1+ T2+ (disease is present), (2) T1+ T2− (negative),
(3) T1− T2+ (negative), and (4) T1− T2− (disease is absent).

(1) Individuals must be positive in both tests to be classified as positive.

(2) Increases specificity but compromises sensitivity.
Sensitivity (net) = Sensitivity T1 × Sensitivity T2.[11]

(3) Specificity (net) = (Specificity T1 + Specificity T2) −
Specificity T1 × Specificity T2.

(4) Appropriate when false-positive causes significant loss
of subjects and is of concern.[11,12]

VI. **Types of Variables, Random Variables, and Probability
Distributions [PHCC.1.2, 1.4]**

A. *Variable* refers to a characteristic of interest in a study that has
different values for different subjects (that which varies).[13]

1. It is the measure of a single characteristic.

2. Termed variable because it varies or changes with subjects.

B. Sources of variation: (1) disease status, (2) biological differences,
(3) measurement conditions, (4) measurement methods,
(5) measurement error, and (6) random error.

1. Statistical methods/tools are used to make sense of the variation in data.

C. Types of variables in public health research: Measurement scales
or type of variable determines which type of statistical method is
appropriate for a given set of data.[14] For example, if a variable
such as weight or blood pressure is measured in a ratio scale,
mean is an appropriate statistical method to summarize the data.

On the other hand, if the scale of measurement is ordinal, median becomes an appropriate method for the summary, as well as frequency distribution (ordinal and nominal).

1. *Nominal (unordered) variables* (naming or categorical) that have no measurement scales (e.g., skin color).
2. *Binary or dichotomous variable* or observation is a nominal measure that has two outcomes [e.g., gender (male → 1, female → 2), survival (yes → 1, no → 0)].
3. *Discrete variables* are binary and nominal, so termed because the categories are separate from each other [e.g., gender (male versus female)].
4. Ordinal *(ordered categories)* variables are those with underlying order to their values [e.g., fatigue scale (0–10), absent, mild, moderate, severe].
5. Continuous or dimensional variables are characteristics that are measured on a continuum (e.g., systolic blood pressure, diastolic blood pressure, height, weight, age, etc.). Compared with ordinal, nominal, or discrete data, continuous variables (interval and ratio) allow for more detailed information and inferences. [PHCC.1.3]

D. *Random variable* refers to a variable in a study in which subjects are randomly selected.[13] For example, if the subjects in a study to examine the survival of men treated for localized prostate cancer with radical prostatectomy are a random sample selected from the larger population, then race and Gleason score are examples of random variables. [PHCC.1.4]

E. *Probability distribution* is used to summarize values of random variable as a form of frequency distribution. [PHCC.1.4]

F. *Types of probability distribution:* [PHCC.1.4]

1. *Binomial* (yes and no) is a discrete probability distribution in which the associated random variable takes only integer values, 0, 1, 2 . . . *n*. It provides the probability that a specified event or outcome occurs in a given number of independent trials.
2. *Poisson* is a discrete distribution applicable, like binomials, when the outcome is the number of times an event occurs.
3. *Normal (Gaussian) distribution (bell-shaped curve)* is a continuous probability distribution. This distribution takes any value;

it is a smooth, bell-shaped curve; and it is symmetric about the mean of the distribution, symbolized by μ, and a standard deviation symbolized by σ.[5]

4. *Standard normal (Z) distribution* refers to the distribution with a mean of 0 and a standard deviation of 1. Mathematically, Z (Z-score, normal deviate, standard score or critical ratio) $= (X - \mu) / \sigma$.[5]

VII. Sampling, Sample Size, and Power [PHCC.1.5]

A. Statistics deals with samples, and the main reason for research is to infer, or generalize, from a sample (sets of observations from one group of subjects) to a larger population (others who are similar to the subjects in the sample).[5,9,13]

B. Statistics is the procedure by which some members of a given population are selected as representatives of the entire population.[6,15]

C. The process of inference requires statistical methods based on probability.

D. Probability of a given outcome is the number of times that outcome occurs divided by the total number of trials.

E. Uses of probability: (1) understanding and interpreting data; (2) indicating how much confidence there is in estimates such as the means, or relative risks; (3) understanding the meaning of *p* values.[9,13]

F. *Probability rules:*

1. *Mutually exclusive events and the additional rule:* Two or more events are mutually exclusive if the occurrence of one precludes the occurrence of the others. The probability is found by adding the probabilities of two events (addition rule) → P(A or B) = P(A) + P(B).[13]

2. *Independent events and multiplication rule:* Two events are independent if the outcome of one event has no effect on the outcome of the second (multiplication rule) → P(A and B) = P(A) × P(B).

G. *Population versus sample:* Population describes a large set or collection of items with common characteristics, whereas sample refers to the subset of the population, selected so as to be representative of the larger population.[16,17]

H. *Why sample? "Bigger is not always better":* (1) Samples are quick to study; (2) they are less expensive; (3) it is difficult or impossible to study the entire population; (4) accuracy of result can be compared with the total population; (5) if properly selected, probability methods can be used to estimate the error in the resulting statistics, making a probability statement about the observations in the study; and (6) samples can be selected to reduce heterogeneity.[6,9,13,16,17]

I. *Sampling techniques:* (1) probability sampling—ensures that a sample will lead to reliable and valid inference, and (2) nonprobability sampling (unknown probability of selection)—deprived of the randomness needed to estimate sampling errors.

J. *Types of probability sampling:* (1) simple random sampling—in which every subject has an equal probability of being selected for the study; (2) systematic sampling—in which every *k*th item is selected, where *k* is determined by number of items in the sampling frame divided by desired sample size; (3) stratified sampling—in which the population is first divided into relevant strata or subgroups, and random sample is then selected from each stratum or subgroup; and (4) cluster sampling—in which the population is divided into clusters and a subset of the clusters is randomly selected.[6,18]

K. *Sampling unit (element):* Subject under observation on which information is collected (e.g., women aged 55 or older undergoing mammography).

L. *Sampling fraction:* ratio between sample size and population size [e.g., 100 out of 4,000 (10%)].

M. *Sampling frame:* list of all sampling units from which sample is drawn (e.g., list of women aged 55 or older undergoing mammography).

N. *Sampling scheme:* method of selecting sampling units from sampling frame (e.g., random selection, convenience sample).

O. *Sample size estimation and power*
   1. *Sample size estimation*
      a. Sample size estimation for descriptive survey—one proportion. Using the formula for one proportion, $n = z^2 \times p \times q / d^2$, where n is the sample size, z is the alpha risk expressed in Z-score, p = the expected prevalence, $q = 1 - p$, and d is the desired/absolute precision.[6,9,13]
      b. Sample size estimation—two proportions or groups. Using the formula, $n = z_1 - \alpha/2[P_1(1 - P_1) + P_2(1 - P_2)] / d^2$, where n = sample size (each group), $z_1 - \alpha/2$ = confidence interval, P_1 = estimated proportion (larger), P_2 = estimated proportion (smaller), and d = desired precision.[6,9,13]

2. *Statistical power*
   a. Probability that the test will reject a false null hypothesis.
   b. Probability that a study will not result in a type II error.
   c. The higher the power, the greater the chance of obtaining a statistically significant result when the null hypothesis is false.
   d. Depends on significance criterion as well as the effect size or the size of the difference.
   e. The power of a test to reject the null hypothesis when indeed the alternative hypothesis is true = $1 - \beta$.[6,19]

Table 1-8   Hypothesis Testing and Relationship Between Type I and Type II Errors

	Null Hypothesis	
Test Results	**False**	**True**
Significant	Power	Type I error
Nonsignificant	Type II error	

VIII. **Research Questions, Hypothesis Testing, and Statistical Inference (Testing) [PHCC.1.6]**
   A. Reading and interpreting scientific research requires understanding how research questions are formulated, hypotheses asserted, and specific test statistics selected to test the hypotheses.
   B. Scientific finding, which commences with hypothesis testing and asserting an association, involves (1) measurement of the magnitude of the outcome effect of interest by comparing outcome between groups with differing exposure, (2) measurement of variation among the observations of interest within exposure groups, (3) measurement of the ratio of outcome effect to variation (e.g., confounding), (4) elimination of alternative explanations (e.g., confounding, bias, random error-chance), and (5) ascertainment of association.[13,20]
   C. *Research question* refers to a statement that identifies the phenomenon to be investigated (e.g., "Does coffee drinking result in pancreatic neoplasm?").

D. Research questions could involve one group of subjects who are measured on one or two occasions. [For example, mean milk consumption and bone density in women 45 years and older. Appropriate research questions: (1) Is the mean milk consumption of women 45 years and older different in our sample compared with the National Study on Nutrition (NSN) sample? In other words, how confident are we that the observed mean milk consumption in our sample is X oz/day? (2) Is the mean bone density (X) in the NSN of women 45 years and older significantly different from our sample?]

E. *What is the hypothesis?* The hypothesis tests or estimates the mean value of a numerical value (e.g., milk consumption, bone density). This hypothesis testing involves the examination of the mean in one group when the observations are normally distributed (e.g., bone density, milk consumption).

F. *Test Statistic: t-test*
   1. *What is the test statistic?* The *t*-distribution is appropriate in performing the test statistics and obtaining the confidence limits.[21]
   2. Simply stated, the single or one-sample *t*-test compares the mean of a single sample to a known population mean.
   3. The purpose of this test (*t*) or student's *t*-test is to answer research questions about means.
   4. The formula for *t*-test is (Statistic − Hypothesized value) / Estimated standard error of the statistic.[6,13]
   5. *Mathematically:* $t = (X - \mu) / (SD / \sqrt{n}) = (X - \mu) / SE$, where X is the observed or sample mean, μ is the hypothesized mean value of the population (true mean in the population), and SE is the standard error of the mean (X).
   6. *Simply,* Mean(x) − Constant (μ) / SD(x), where SD(x) is the sum $\{(x_i - \text{Mean}(x))\}^2 / (n - 1)$.[9,13]
   7. To find out whether the observed mean is real [i.e, the observed mean is different from the mean of the NSN, termed the norm or population mean] and not just a random occurrence, the following factors need to be considered: (1) the difference between the observed mean and the norm (NSN) or population mean, implying much larger or smaller—magnitude of the mean difference → greater difference; (2) the amount of variability among subjects, implying

less variation—smaller standard deviation in the sample (i.e., homogeneous sample and relatively precise method of measurement); and (3) the number of subjects in the study, implying larger rather than smaller sample.

   a. *Vignette:* Consider a study conducted to compare the mean vitamin C intake among 8th-grade schoolchildren at New School, Texas, with the population mean (Texas Study of Nutrition). If the investigator found a greater SD, what is the probable explanation?

   b. *Solution:* If the SD is greater in the sample studied (8th-grade children at New School), it is likely that (1) vitamin C intake varies widely from one child to another, or (2) a crude measure devise is used to ascertain the vitamin C intake (improper, imprecise, or crude measure).

BOX 1-5   STUDENT *t*-TEST

- The *t*-test is an appropriate statistical test that compares the means of two groups of observations.
- Each group is assumed to be a sample from a distinct population, and the responses in each group are independent of those in the other group.
- The observations should be randomly assigned to the two groups, so that any difference in response is due to the treatment and not to other factors.
- The paired *t*-test compares two paired groups so one can make inferences about the size of the average treatment effect, implying the average difference between the paired measurements.
- The rationale for using a paired *t*-test is to control for experimental variability as well as potential non-normality of the response.
- Thus by analyzing only the differences, a paired *t*-test corrects for those sources of scatter or variability.

---

  8. *Assumptions:*

   a. Normal distribution.

   b. If normality is not assumed, observations should be more than 30 subjects; thus means become normally distributed above this number regardless of the distribution of original observations (central limit theorem).

    c. Even with violation of normal distribution, a *t*-test could still be performed because it is robust for nonnormal data, implying the drawing of a proper conclusion even when the assumptions are not met, including normality.

BOX 1-6   APPLICATION OF DEGREE OF FREEDOM AND *t*-TEST TECHNIQUE

- When the population standard deviation is unknown and the sample size is less than 30 ($n < 30$), the distribution of the test statistic cannot be guaranteed to be normal.
- Hence, the test statistic can be said to conform to a *t* distribution.
- The *t* distribution is similar to the standard normal distribution in that it is symmetrically distributed around a mean value.
- However, the *t* distribution varies from the standard normal, in that its standard deviation is determined by the number of degrees of freedom.
- Degrees of freedom (DF) are calculated from the size of the sample.
- Simply, DF is a measure of the amount of information from the sample data that has been utilized.
- Thus whenever a paired *t*-test statistic is calculated from a sample, one degree of freedom is used up.

---

    9. *Interpretation:* The null hypothesis assumes the equality of means; a significant result at significance level < 0.05) is indicative of the significant difference between the sample mean (X) and the population mean (μ). A nonsignificant mean difference implies that the difference may be due to random error or chance, given the significance level ($p > 0.05$); it does not mean that the two means are equal.[9,13] Simply, it is not possible to be confident about accepting the observed difference because this might be due to random occurrence. [PHCC.1.7]

  G. *Types of t-test* [PHCC.1.6]

    1. *An independent samples t-test* compares the means of two samples, with the assumptions that (a) two groups being compared should be independent of each other, (b) the scores should be normally distributed, (c) dependency must be

measured on an interval or ratio scale, and (d) the independent sample should have only two discrete levels.

BOX 1-7   TWO SAMPLE *t*-TEST

■ The unpaired *t*-test, two sample *t*-test, or independent-samples *t*-test compares the means of two groups, assuming that data are sampled from Gaussian populations (normal distribution).

■ If the *p* value is small (< 0.05), for instance, then it is unlikely that the observed difference is due to random variability or sampling error.

---

2. *A paired samples t-test (dependent t-test or t-test for correlated data)* compares the means of two scores from related samples, with the assumptions that (a) both variables are at interval or ratio scales; (b) both are normally distributed; (c) both are measured with the same scale; and (d) if different scales are involved, the scores should be converted to *Z*-scores prior to *t*-test analysis.

Table 1-9   Comparison Between Standard Normal Distribution (Z-score) and t-Distribution

Test	Description
Z-score	Symmetric with mean of 0 and SE $= 1.0$
	Narrower and lower in tails compared to *t*-distribution. Why? Smaller SE.
t-distribution	Symmetric with mean of 0 and SE > 1.0
	Degree of freedom (df) is $n - 1$.
	Wider and higher in tails compared to *Z*. Why? Larger SD.

---

3. Difference between *t* and *Z* is very small when $n > 30$ subjects.
4. As sample size increases, degree of freedom (df) increases, and the *t*-distribution becomes almost the same as *Z*.
5. With $n > 30$, either of the two distributions can be used.
6. *Other statistic for mean differences:* Because using a *t*-test involves a normal distribution and $n > 30$, another statistic

for evaluating mean differences when these assumptions are not met is the Wilcoxon sign rank test (Mann-Whitney test), which is adequate for paired design as well as one sample.

7. Hypothesis testing about the proportion is performed using the *Z*-distribution.

    a. The process involves a research question [e.g., Is there a significant difference in the observed proportion (0.20) of children with moderate to high physical activity in a sample, compared with the population proportion of 0.40?]

8. Comparing two independent proportions involves the use of a *Z*-test.

9. Comparing frequencies of proportion in two groups can be achieved with the chi-square test of independence.

10. Like the *t*-test, it is *Z*-approximation (approximate test).

11. It is based on a null hypothesis of no difference/relationship/association or dependency.

12. A nonparametric procedure: [PHCC.1.5, 1.6, 1.7]

    a. Research questions: (1) Is there difference in the proportion of older men treated for prostate problems who received hormonal therapy relative to those who did not receive hormonal therapy? (2) Is there an association or relationship between women with autoimmune disorder and race?

    b. *Hypothesis* (test the equality of these two proportions): The null hypothesis for dependency is that there is no racial difference among women with autoimmune disorders or simply, women with autoimmune disorder do not differ by race.

    c. *Mathematically:* $(\chi^2 = (O - E)^2 / E)$, where O is the observed frequency, E = the expected frequency → $\chi^2_{(df)} = \Sigma$(Observed frequency − Expected frequency) / Expected frequency.[6,9,13,22,23]

    d. If no relationship exists, the observed frequencies will be very close to the expected frequency, thus rendering the chi-square value small.

    e. If more than 20% of expected, not the observed frequency, is < 5 → Fisher's exact test.[9,13]

f. *Assumption* (same as one sample *t*-test): (1) The expected frequency for each category should be at least 1. (2) No more than 20% of the categories should have expected frequencies of < 5.

g. *Test statistic:* Chi-square test of independence.

BOX 1-8   CHI-SQUARE NON-PARAMETRIC TEST

- The chi-square statistic is a non-parametric analytic method used to compare the observed frequency of some observation with an expected frequency.
- The comparison of observed and expected frequencies is used to calculate the value of the chi-square statistic, which in turn can be compared with the distribution of chi-square to make an inference about a statistical issue such as the relationship between pet ownership and depressive symptoms, hypertension and sodium intake, maternal preconception weight and low birth weight, etc.

---

h. *Interpretation:* A significant chi-square test implies that two variables are not independent, meaning that there is an association between the two variables, whereas a non-significant result indicates that the variables do not vary significantly from independence.[5,9]

13. *Vignette:* Consider a study conducted to assess the relationship between gender and cardiomyopathies among U.S. residents. If the investigators found that men were 68% with cardiomyopathies while women were 40%, and the significance level was < 0.05, with a $\chi^2 = 27.32$, and df = 1, will you consider this finding to indicate that men are significantly more likely to have cardiomyopathies relative to women?

a. *Solution:* With the chi-square value (27.32), which is large, given 1 degree of freedom (3.84 critical value), and the *p* value, < 0.05, there is a significant association between gender and cardiomyopathies, leading to the rejection of the null hypothesis of independence or no association. Therefore, the conclusion drawn is accurate:

men are more likely to have cardiomyopathies compared with women, based on the proportion in the result of the investigation.

   b. *Analysis of variance:* Comparison of means in three or more groups involves the use of analysis of variance (ANOVA)—univariate or one-way ANOVA.

   c. *Assumptions:* (1) group independence (if subjects belong to more than one group → repeated measures ANOVA); (2) one independent variable (if more than one independent variable → factorial ANOVA (two-way ANOVA); (3) dependent variable is at interval or ratio levels, and is *normally distributed* → *parametric procedure*; (4) population variance is the same in each group (homogeneity of variance); and (5) observations are a random sample.[24]

   d. The test statistic for ANOVA (*F*-test) is not influenced by moderate departure from the assumption of normality, especially with large number of observations—*robust*.

   e. Extremely skewed observations → Kruskal-Wallis test (nonparametric procedure).

   f. Serious violation of ANOVA assumptions, as in *t*-test assumptions violation → Wilcoxon rank sum test (nonparametric procedure) for one-way ANOVA and Friedman test for one-way repeated measures ANOVA and two-way ANOVA (nonparametric procedure).[22]

14. *Statistic: F*-test for two variances: ratio of the variance among means to the variance among subjects within each group.[5,23,25]

15. *Hypothesis:* The null hypothesis is that the two variances are equal (i.e., the variation among means is not much greater than the variation among individual observations within any given group).[9,22,23]

16. *Interpretation:* The *F*-value, degrees of freedom, and the significance level are necessary for the conclusion to be drawn on the significant mean differences between the groups.[5,9]

17. Comparison of means in three or more groups with a covariate that is confounding involves the use of covariates (ANCOVA).

18. ANCOVA serves as a method of controlling for confounding.[22,23]

BOX 1-9   STATISTICAL TECHNIQUES RATIONALE

- An *unpaired t-test* is appropriate in testing the hypothesis comparing two groups that consist of different individuals and the measurement scale is interval and drawn from normally distributed populations.
- *Chi-square* is appropriate in testing the hypothesis of group independence when the measurement scale is either binary or categorical.
- *Logistic regression* technique is adequate in predicting the effect of the explanatory variable on outcome if the outcome is measured in a continuous scale and the explanatory or independent on a mixed scale.

IX. **Analysis Techniques for Epidemiologic Data**
    [PHCC.1.5, 1.6, 1.7, 1.8]
    A. Various test statistics are available for analyzing the relationship between two or more variables.
    B. The selection of a test or statistic [e.g., *t*-test (testing for statistical significance)] depends on (1) the scale of the measurement of the dependent and independent variables, parametric (continuous scale data), or nonparametric (nominal/discrete scale data) distribution; (2) the type of design (before and after comparison); and (3) the sampling procedure (random sampling), among other factors.[14]
    C. *Bivariate* or *univariable* analysis refers to the analysis of the relationship between *one* independent (X) and *one* dependent variable (Y). For example, if an investigator decides to examine the relationship between height and weight of 100 high school students, he or she may wish to determine if weight (Y) depends on height (X).[18,24]
    D. *Multivariable analysis* refers to the analysis between a single dependent variable and more than one independent variable (e.g., a study to determine the impact of race and gender in the development of colorectal cancer). The independent variables are age (X_1) and race (X_2), while the dependent variable is colorectal cancer (Y).
    E. *Multivariate analysis* is the technique that involves more than one dependent and more than a single independent variable.[9,13,25] This term is *not* interchangeable with multivariable analysis, and it is often used incorrectly.

Table 1-10 Analysis of Research Questions About Relationships Among Variables: Correlation			
Statistical Method	**Variable**	**Assumption**	**Statistic**
Correlation: Pearson	Dependent (outcome, response) and independent (predictors, explanatory) must be measured in continuous scale	1. Random sample 2. Bivariate normal distribution	Pearson product moment correlation coefficient (r)
Correlation: Spearman's rho/ Kendall tau	1. Numerical variables that are not normally distributed 2. Ordinal variables	1. Rank order data 2. Ordinal data, or interval or ratio 3. Nonparametric data	Spearman's rho or rank correlation (r)

F. *Correlation analysis*

1. If either of the two variables is not normally distributed, Pearson correlation is considered inappropriate.[14,24]

   a. *Alternate approach to analysis:* (1) Either one or both variables should be transformed to achieve near normal distribution. (2) Spearman rank correlation, which is a nonparametric test, should be used.

BOX 1-10   CORRELATION ANALYSIS & SIMPLE LINEAR REGRESSION

- *Correlation analysis* is conducted to determine whether or not there is a relationship or an association. A significant positive correlation suggests that the relationship is directly proportional, meaning that Y (response variable-systolic pressure) increases as X (independent variable-alcohol consumption) increases.

- A *simple linear regression* is conducted to examine a straight line relationship between an independent variable, X (measured in a continuous or binary scale) and a response variable Y (measured in a continuous scale).

---

2. *Interpretation:* (1) correlation coefficient, r, is between -1.0 and $+1.0$, with r close to 0.0 considered to be a weak relationship;

(2) 1.0 or -1.0 = strong relationship; (3) > 0.7 = strong corre-lation; (4) 0.3 to 0.7 = moderate correlation; (5) < 0.3 = weak correlation.[3,14,24]

G. *Linear regression (least square regression) analysis*

1. Refers to a regression method that is based on the least squares method:

    a. Linear regression is an analytic technique used to predict the value of one characteristic or variable (Y) from knowledge of the other (X). The regression equation is given by $Y = \beta_0 + \beta_1 X + \epsilon$.

    b. It is termed *linear* because this method, unlike correlation, measures only a straight line or linear relationship between two variables (simple linear regression).

    c. The least squares method minimizes the differences between the actual value of Y and the predicted value of $Y\{\Sigma(Y - \acute{Y})^2\}$, which is measured by the error term ϵ $(Y - \acute{Y})$ in the regression equation (G-1-a)[9,13,25] *(please see the regression equation above)*.

2. In *simple linear regression* (SLR), only a single independent or explanatory variable (X) is used to predict the outcome (Y).

3. *Multiple linear regression* (MLR), refers to a regression technique that, like the SLR, is based on the least squares method, where more than one independent variable is included in the prediction equation.

    a. *Mathematically:* $Y = \beta_0 + \beta_1 X_1 + \beta_2 X_2....\beta_i X_i$, with β_0 and $\beta_1...\beta_i$ as the regression parameters.

4. *Interpretation:* The SLR equation is given by $Y = \beta_0 + \beta_1 X + \epsilon$, where β_1 is the slope or the regression coefficient; β_0 is the intercept of the regression line (β_1 and β_0 are the population parameters); and ϵ is the error term, which is the distance the actual value of Y depart from the regression line.

5. *R square (R^2)* in the linear regression model output is the coefficient of determination that measures the proportion of the variance of the dependent variable (Y) that can be explained by the variation in the independent variable (X).

6. *The standard error of estimate* (model output) measures the dispersion for the prediction equation.

7. *Test statistics:* (1) ANOVA in the model uses *F*-statistic to determine the statistical significance of the regression equation and (2) the *t*-statistic test, whether or not the regression coefficient is statistically significant.[25]

Table 1-11 Analysis of Research Questions About Relationships Among Variables: Linear Regression			
Statistical Method*	**Variable**	**Assumption**	**Statistic**
Simple linear regression (SLR)	1. Response is measured in continuous scale 2. Independent may be in continuous or binary scale	1. Both variables are interval or ratio scaled 2. Dependent (*Y*) must be normally distributed along the predicted line (homogeneity) 3. Relationship is linear	Regression statistic: (1) *t*-statistic (2) *F*-statistic
Multiple linear regression	Same as SLR; more than single dependent variables	Same as SLR; variables are also related to each other linearly	Same as SLR

*Performs the statistical test to determine the likelihood of any observed relationship between *X* and *Y* variables.

H. *Other types of regression (multiple)*
    1. *Polynomial regression* refers to multiple regression, in which each term in the equation is a power of *X*.[24]
    2. *Discriminant analysis* predicts group membership with only two groups and uses continuous independent variables only. *Log-linear analysis* focuses on the analysis of the conditional relationship of two or more categorical values; unlike binomial logistic regression, the dependent variable is categorical and the link function is the log (log of the dependent variable), not logit, and the predictions are estimates of the cell counts in contingency table, not the logit of the dependent variable, *y*.[26,27]

I. *Logistic regression (LR) (binomial or ordinary)*

1. Logistic regression is a form of regression analysis (logit transformation) in which the outcome is binary and the independent variables could be measured in mixed scales (categorical, binary, mixed continuous, and categorical).[28]

2. Logit transformation (logit p) for the binary outcome or dependent variable is denoted by $\ln[p / (1 - p)]$, where the logit transformation takes any value from minus infinity to plus infinity.[9,13]

3. This method calculates the probability or success over the probability of failure, thus presenting the odds ratio as the final result [e.g., logistic regression is used in determining the probability of developing prostate cancer, given exposure to organophosphates (pesticides) after adjusting for other known and postulated risk factors].

   a. Classified under generalized linear model.

   b. Also, the dependent variable can have more than two levels (e.g., multinomial and polytomous logistic regression).

4. Like SLR or MLR, logistic regression is a predictive model and is used to predict the outcome or dependent variable on the basis of continuous and/or binary/categorical independent or predictor/explanatory variables, as well as to determine the percent variance of the dependent variable that is explained by the independents, rank the relative importance of independents, assess the interaction effects, and control for confounding in the multivariable model.

5. This method uses maximum likelihood estimation after transforming the dependent variable into a logit variable, implying obtaining the natural log of the odds of the outcome or dependent variable occurring or not occurring—the probability of the outcome occurring.

6. The goal of this method is to correctly predict the outcome of the individual cases using the most parsimonious model.

7. Unlike the SLR, the relationship between the predictor and the response variables is not a linear function, but a logit transformation of the outcome variable.

8. The changes in the log odds of the outcome are estimated and not the changes in the dependent or outcome variable itself.

9. *Mathematically:* $\theta = e^{(\alpha + \beta_1 X_1 + \beta_2 X_2 + \ldots + \beta_i X_i)} / 1 + e^{(\alpha + \beta_1 X_1 + \beta_2 X_2 + \ldots + \beta_i X_i)}$, where α is the constant of the equation and β is the coefficient of the predictor or independent variables in the model.[28]

10. Given the probability of success (p) of a binomial outcome variable (y), the logistic regression model is: Logit (p) = $\ln(p / 1 - p)$ = alpha + beta$_1$ x$_1$ + beta$_2$X$_2$ . . . beta$_k$X$_k$.

11. Likewise, solving for $p = e^{(\alpha + \beta_1 X_1 + \beta_2 X_2 + \ldots + \beta_i X_i)} / 1 + e^{(\alpha + \beta_1 X_1 + \beta_2 X_2 + \ldots + \beta_i X_i)}$.[28,29]

12. The occurrence of outcome in this model is an exponential function of the independent variables: $Px = 1 / \{1 + \exp[-(b_0 + b_1 x_1 + b_2 x_2 + b_3 x_3 + b_4 x_4 \ldots b_i x_i)]\}$, where b_0 is the intercept (constant), b_1, b_3, b_3, b_4, . . . b_i are the regression coefficient, while exp represents the base of the natural logarithm (2.718).

13. *Mathematically,* the odds ratio in logistic regression can be computed from the coefficient of regression $\beta \rightarrow OR = e^\beta$, where exp = 2.718.

14. The Wald statistic (test) tests the statistical significance of the individual independent variable [each coefficient (β)] in the model.

15. The Wald test is a squared Z-test with chi-square distribution: $Z = \beta / SE$ [Coefficient (β) / Standard error (SE)]. This is the squared ratio of the unstandardized logit coefficient to its SE.

16. *Wald statistic interpretation:* Some statisticians have suggested that large logit increases SEs, lowering the Wald statistic, thus leading to a type II error implying a false-negative, assuming that the effect is not significant, which indeed it is (rejecting the alternate hypothesis of difference).

17. *Model testing (appropriateness of the model):* Goodness-of-fit (Hosmer-Lemeshow), which is a chi-square statistic with a desirable outcome of nonsignificance, indicates that the model prediction does not significantly differ from the observed.[28]

18. *Model testing (backward stepwise elimination):* Likelihood-ratio test (LRT) uses the ratio of the maximized value of the likelihood function of the full model (L_1) over the maximized value of the likelihood function for the simpler model such as the model without predictors and or interaction (L_0). *Mathematically:* LRT = $-2\log (L_0 / L_1) = -2\{\log(L_0) - \log(L_1)\} = -2(L_0 - L_1)$.[9,29]

19. The reduced model could be a baseline model or initial model with constant only, thus termed a null model. The full model then becomes the model with the predictors.

   a. An LRT can then test the difference between the initial or null model, model with constant only, and the model with the coefficients from the predictors.

   b. The model is significant at $P < 0.05$, indicating that the fitted model is significantly different from the null model or model chi-square test as it is termed.

   c. This model does not ensure that every independent variable in the model is significant.

   d. Best model—the final model, which implies that adding another variable would not improve the model significantly (e.g., model with and without interaction).

Table 1-12 Analysis of Research Questions About Relationships Among Variables: Logistic Regression			
Statistical Method*	**Variable**	**Assumption**	**Statistic**
Logistic regression: unconditional (ULR)	*Outcome* is binary *Independent* variables are categorical and categorical and continuous (mixed)	Does not assume linear relationship Outcome need not be normally distributed Outcome need not be homoscedastic for level of predictors No normally distributed error term	Wald statistic (β) Hosmer–Lemeshow (χ^2) (goodness of fit) Likelihood ratio test (overall model)
Logistic regression: conditional	Same as ULR; matched pairs $(1 - K)*$	Same as ULR	Same as ULR

*Matching tends to increase the degrees of freedom relative to the cases. A better approach to the analysis is conditional logistic regression, which maximizes the likelihood estimate in logistic regression.

20. *Interpretation of logistic regression result* (OR = e^β): The odds in favor of success for a subject (*A*) (exposure = 1) are given by $OR_A = P_A / (1 - P_A)$, and the odds in favor of success for a subject (*B*) (exposure = 0) are given by $OR_B = P_B / (1 - P_B)$. The odds ratio is then (OR) = OR_A / OR_B.

21. The odds ratio relates a disease or outcome to the '*i*'th exposure for two hypothetical subjects *A* and *B*, where *A* is exposed and *B* is not.

    a. In the multivariable model, this odds ratio relates disease to the '*i*'th exposure variable, controlling for the levels of all other exposure variables in the model.

J. *Types of generalized linear models (counts data):* Poisson regression, negative binomial regression, and zero-inflated regression models are appropriate for the analysis of count data that are: (1) highly nonnormally distributed and (2) not well estimated by ordinary least squares regression.

Table 1-13 Statistical Methods Involving Counts Data	
Statistical Method	**Description and Applications**
Poisson regression	To model the number of occurrences of an event of interest or the rate of occurrence of an event of interest, as a function of some independent variables
	Efficient when the dependent variable is a count variable—with same length of observation time (e.g., number of days absent from work)
	Incidence rate ratio is the point estimate
Negative binomial regression	Used to estimate count models when the Poisson model is inappropriate due to overdispersion (which is most of the time)
	In Poisson distribution the mean and variance are equal; thus, when the variance is greater than the mean, the distribution is said to display overdispersion; if lower than the mean, underdispersion
	When there is overdispersion, the Poisson estimates are inefficient with standard errors biased downward, yielding spuriously large Z-values
	Efficient for dispersed count data, as an extension of generalized Poisson regression
Zero-inflated Poisson (ZIP) regression model	Extension of generalized Poisson regression with count data having extra zeros
	ZIP is useful to analyze such data
	Efficient where overdispersion is assumed to be caused by an excessive number of zeros

K. *Statistical analysis method for event data (survival analysis)*

1. This method involves *censored observations* or data, where subjects have been observed unequal lengths of time and the outcome is not yet known for all subjects: left-censored if the episode started before the period of observation and right-censored if the episode ended after the period of observation.[30,31]

    a. Assesses the effect of independent variables on the event (what terminates an episode such as death in a clinical trial of drug or other therapeutics) in question.

    b. Simply, survival analysis assesses the simultaneous effect of several variables (covariates) on length of survival.

2. Time to event analysis or duration modeling is (a) parametric, where the shape of the baseline hazard function is assumed (e.g., Weilbull model); or (b) semi-parametric, where there is no assumption of the baseline hazard function shape but focus is on predicting the hazard ratio (HR) (e.g., Cox regression or proportional hazard model).[31,32]

3. *Proportional hazard model (Cox regression)* refers to the HR remaining constant over time, which does not mean the *same* over time as often misinterpreted. Cox regression: Hazard rate (not survival time) is the function of the independent covariates $H(t) = H0(t) \times \exp(b_1X_1 + b_2X_2 + b_3X_3 + \ldots\ldots + b_mX_m)$; $X_1..X_m$ are predictor variables or covariates and $H0(t)$ is the baseline hazard at time t.
    Hazard ratio $- \ln[(H(t) / H0(t)] = b_1X_1 + b_2X_2 + b_3X_3 + \ldots\ldots + b_mX_m$. $H(t) / H(0)t = HR$. Hazard is the probability of the endpoint, death.
    Assumptions: (i) *Proportionality*—Given 2 observations with different values for the independent variables, the ratio of the hazard functions for these two observations does not depend on time. (ii) *Log-linearity*—There is a log-linear relationship between the independent variables and the underlying hazard function.

    a. This is Cox regression assumption: violation that may either overestimate or underestimate the point estimate (HR).

4. *Hazard, hazard rates, and ratios*

    a. *Hazard* is the event of interest occurring (e.g., death or biochemical failure in a clinical trial of a therapeutic agent).

      b. *Hazard rate* at a given time is the probability of the event given that the dependent = 1, occurring in that time period, given survival through all prior time intervals.

      c. *Hazard ratio*, also termed hazard function, refers to the estimate of the ratio of the hazard rate in group *A* (treatment group) to the hazard rate in group *B* (placebo group).

5. The survival function [S(*t*)] is the cumulative frequency of the proportion of the sample not experiencing the event by time *t* (alive or surviving observations).

      a. *Mathematically:* $S(t) = 1 - F(t)$, which is the probability that the event will not occur until time *t*, which also implies the proportion of participants surviving beyond any given time *t*.[30,32]

6. The *survival function plot* enables the comparison of the survival rates of two or more groups in a study.

_OX 1-11   EQUALITY OF SURVIVAL & LOG RANK TEST

- Two or more life table curves could be tested to determine if they are significantly different.
- The *z*-test for proportion is used for the actuarial curves while the log-rank test is used for Kaplan-Meier curves.
- The log rank test is an approximate chi-square test, and compares the number of observed deaths in each group with the number of deaths that would be expected from the number of deaths in the combined groups, implying if group membership or distinction did not matter.
- The log-rank test is also referred to as Cox-Mantel log-rank statistic, Mantel log-rank statistic.
- The log-rank test, as may be incorrectly interpreted, does not involve ranking nor does it employ logarithm in its computation of the survival differences.

---

7. *Statistic:* (a) LRT for the model (sometimes *score statistic* is used), (b) regression coefficients (β) for the statistical significance of individual independent variables or covariates in the model, and (c) log-rank test for the equality of survival function.

8. *Interpretation:* Hazard ratio (HR), sometimes termed odds ratio, is given by exponent (β). If HR = 1.0, this means that

the covariate (e.g., androgen deprivation therapy, or ADT in the model) has no effect or influence on the time to event for the status or dependent variable (e.g., death from prostate cancer). If HR > 1.0, this indicates the increases in the odds of dying given the use of ADT. Inversely, if HR < 1.0, this means that ADT diminishes or decreases the odds of dying on the subjects placed on ADT relative to those who are not.

9. *Survival curves estimation:* Kaplan-Meier survival analysis, also termed *product-limit method*, refers to a nonparametric method of generating tables and plots or graphs of survival, failure, or hazards functions for time to event data. (a) The assumption of the method is that the event must be dependent on time. (b) It involves the plotting of survival function on linear scale. (c) It is not designed to assess the effect or influence of covariates on the time to event status variable. Success or effectiveness of treatment is measured in terms of time that some desirable outcome is maintained. Such analysis (time-related patterns of survival) techniques originated from the life table procedures. Kaplan-Meier, also termed the product limit method, is more commonly used in biomedical and public health research compared to the actuarial method. Kaplan-Meier product limit and actuarial methods are commonly used to estimate survival experience of samples. Both methods are similar except that time since entry in the study is not divided into intervals for analysis in the Kaplan-Meier product limit method. Two or more life table curves could be tested to determine if they are significantly different. The Z-test for proportion is used for the actuarial curves while the log-rank test is used for Kaplan-Meier curves. The log-rank test is an approximate chi-square test and compares the number of observed deaths in each group with the number of deaths that would be expected from the number of deaths in the combined groups, implying that group membership or distinction did not matter. The log-rank test is also referred to as the Cox-Mantel log-rank statistic or the Mantel log-rank statistic. The log-rank test, as may be incorrectly interpreted, does not involve ranking, nor

does it employ logarithm in its computation of the survival differences of two or more groups.[33]

X. **Critique of Scientific Literature—Interpreting Statistics in Public Health Research [PHCC.1.8, 1.9, 1.10]**

A. *Study designs:* Determine the study design to address the research questions: (1) experimental (clinical trial, therapeutic, parallel, preventive, community, individual, etc.) and (2) observational (ecologic, cross-sectional, case-control, cohort, etc.).

B. *Scale of measurement* [PHCC 1.2, 1.3]

1. Determine the scale of measurement of the variables (nominal, categorical, discrete, ratio, interval) for the dependent and independent variables.

2. Determine if data presented are assumed to follow normal distribution or not, parametric or nonparametric.

3. If data are assumed to be normally distributed, is the descriptive statistics appropriate (mean, standard deviation, standard error, etc.)?

4. If data are assumed to be nonparametric, is the descriptive statistics presented in terms of proportions, percentages?

C. *Internal validity* (random error, bias, and confounding) refers to accurate measurement of study effects without bias—this bias presents threats to the internal validity of the study. Thus to claim internal validity, a study must be capable of producing unbiased inferences regarding the target population, implying inferences beyond the study population. The precision and accuracy of measurement are essential to study validity. Whereas precision refers to the degree to which a variable has nearly the same value when measured several times, accuracy pertains to the degree to which a variable actually represents what it is supposed to represent or measure. Precision may be enhanced by (1) repetition; (2) refinement; (3) observer's training and performance verification; (4) standardization; and (5) automation, which minimizes variability due to observers. Accuracy may be improved by (1) specific markers and better instruments, (2) unobtrusive measurement, (3) blinding, and (4) instrument calibration.

D. *Role of random error:* Assuming a random sample was taken from the population studied, is this sample representative of the population? Is the observed result influenced by sampling variability? Is there a recognizable source of error such as quality of questions, faulty instrument, etc.? Is the error due to chance, given no connection to recognizable source or error? Random error can be minimized by (1) improving design, (2) enlarging sample size, and (3) increasing precision, as well as by using good quality control during study implementation.

E. The null hypothesis states that there is no association between the exposure and the disease variables, which in most instances translates to the statement that the ratio measure of association = 1.0 (null), with the alternate hypothesis stated to contradict the null (one-tail or two-tail)—that the measure of association is not equal to 1.0.

F. *Significance level (alpha):* The test statistics that depend on the design as well as the measure of the outcome and independent variables yield a p value. The p value (significance level) is the probability of obtaining the observed result and more extreme results by chance alone, given that the null hypothesis is true. The significance level is arbitrary cutoff at 5% (0.05). A $p < 0.05$ is considered statistically significant, implying that the null hypothesis of no association should be rejected in favor of the alternate hypothesis. Simply, this is indicative of the fact that random error is an unlikely explanation of the observed result or point estimate (statistically significant). With $p > 0.05$, the null hypothesis should not be rejected, which implies that the observed result may be explained by random error or sampling variability (statistically nonsignificant).

1. *Vignette:* Consider a study to examine the association between physical inactivity and BMI among school-age children. Assume that the investigators found the risk of obesity (BMI > 30 kg/m^2) was 4 times higher among children with low levels of physical activity, and the p associated with the relative risk is 0.03. What is the possible explanation of this result, and is this result statistically significant?

2. *Solution:* (1) This simply means that if the null hypothesis is true; there is a 3% probability of obtaining the observed

result or one or more extreme (RR = 4.0 or greater) by chance alone. (2) Because the p is < 0.05, the observed result is statistically significant.

G. *Type I or alpha error* refers to incorrect rejection of the null hypothesis, implying the rejection of the null hypothesis when indeed the null hypothesis is true.

1. When the null hypothesis is true and the investigator rejects the null hypothesis, type I error is committed (false-positive).

H. *Type II or beta error* refers to erroneously failing to reject the null hypothesis when indeed it is false.

1. When the investigator fails to reject the null hypothesis when it is false, type II error is committed (false-negative).

Table 1-14 Hypothesis Testing and Type I Error		
Truth	**No Association**	**Association**
No Association	Correct	Type II error
Association	Type I error*	Correct

*P value is the probability of type I error. Because samples come from the population, the p value plays a role in inferential statistics by allowing conclusions to be drawn regarding the population.

I. *Confidence interval*

1. CI is determined by quantification of precision or random error around the point estimate, with the width of CI determined by random error arising from measurement error or imprecise measurement and sampling variability, and some cutoff value (95%).

2. CI simply implies that if a study were repeated 100 times and 100 point estimates and 100 CIs were estimated, 95 out of 100 CIs will contain the true point estimate (measure of association).

3. CI is used to determine statistical significance of an association. If the 95% fails to include 1.0 (null), then the association is considered to be statistically significant.

BOX 1-12   STANDARD ERROR (SE)

- SE allows the investigator to estimate the probable amount of error the quantitative assertions, as well as enables the performance of statistical significance test (95% Confidence Interval).
- The standard error is calculated using the formula: $SE = SD / \sqrt{n}$, where N is the number of observations.
- For example, if SD = 11.3 and n = 36, substituting: $11.3 / 6 = 1.88$ mm/Hg.
- The larger the sample size (n), the smaller the standard error and the better the estimate of the population mean will be.
- Since SE can be converted to SD and vice versa, SD and SE are both acceptable measures of the amount of errors around the quantitative assertions.

---

4. *Vignette:* Consider a study conducted to examine the role of passive smoking on lung carcinoma, if the 95% CI = 1.4 − 1.9, can we claim that there is a statistically significant association between passive smoking and lung carcinoma?

   a. *Solution:* Because the point estimate for the association lies within the upper and lower confidence limits, and 1.0 is not included, the observed result is statistically significant.

J. *Bias (systematic error) and sources of bias*

   1. Determine if bias, which is systematic error, contributes to the observed results.

   2. *Types of bias:* selection bias, prevalence or incidence bias (admission rate bias—Berkson's fallacy studying hospitalized patients as cases), nonresponse and volunteer bias, etc.

   3. Measurement validity may introduce recall bias, detection bias, information bias, and compliance bias.

   4. Systematic error is likely to occur due to observer bias, subject bias, or instrument bias.

   5. Systematic errors are minimized by improving design and increasing accuracy.

K. *Randomization and blinding (experimental and clinical trial)*

   1. Was randomization properly achieved?

   2. Was double blinding utilized?

L. *Power (rejecting a false alternative hypothesis) and sample size*

   1. Power measures the ability of the test to correctly reject the null hypothesis when the alternative hypothesis is true.

      a. *Mathematically:* Statistical power of a test = 1 − beta.

2. Both alpha and beta errors are involved in sample size computation of a study. Lowering alpha decreases power because it makes it less likely to reject the null hypothesis, even where true differences exist.

BOX 1-13   STATISTICAL SIGNIFICANCE AND TYPE 1 ERROR

- The level at which a result is considered significant is known as the type I error rate or α.
- A p value is a measure of how much evidence one has against the null hypothesis.
- The smaller the p value, the more evidence one has.
- One may combine the p value with the significance level to make a decision on a given test of hypothesis.
- A p value is not the probability that the null hypothesis is true but should be seen as the measure of the strength of the evidence provided by the data in favor of the null hypothesis.

---

3. A small number is unlikely to show the difference between the two groups. Smaller sample sizes reduce power because the translation of sigma into SE of the mean produces a larger SE for smaller samples.

BOX 1-14   SAMPLE SIZE ESTIMATION AND POWER

- **Descriptive Survey:** Using the formula for one proportion: $n = z^2 \times p \times q / d^2$, where n is the sample size, z is the alpha risk expressed in z-score, $p =$ the expected prevalence and $q = 1 - p$, and d is the absolute precision.
- **Two proportions or groups:** Using the formula: $n = z_1 - \alpha/2 \ [P_1 (1 - P_1) + P_2 (1 - P_2)] / d^2$, where $n =$ sample size (each group), $z_1 - \alpha/2 =$ Confidence interval, $P_1 =$ estimated proportion (larger), $P_2 =$ estimated proportion (smaller), and $d =$ desired precision.
- **POWER of** affixed level test against a particular alternative hypothesis is the complement of the probability of a type II error for that alternative hypothesis. The Power of a test is therefore the probability that a fixed level alpha significance test will reject the null hypothesis when a particular value of the parameter is true or correct.
- **Power = 1 − Type II error**

4. Sample size varies with the magnitude of the outcome effect expected. Thus, when variance is large, the outcome effect, even if robust, will be obscured by the underlying variation. Conversely, when the variation is modest, even modest effect may be perceived clearly with a small sample size.

Table 1-15   Choice of Statistical Test for Selected Data

Data Distribution	Groups (number)	Test Statistic— Independent	Test Statistic— Paired
Continuous (nonnormal)	2	Mann-Whitney U test	Wilcoxon signed-ranked test
Continuous (normal)	2 ($n > 30$)	t-test	Paired t-test
Normal (nonnormal)	≥ 3	Kruskal-Wallis test	Friedman test
Normal (normal)	≥ 3	ANOVA	Repeated measures ANOVA
Ordinal	2	Mann-Whitney U test	Wilcoxon signed-ranked test
	≥ 3	Kruskal-Wallis test	Friedman test
Nominal	2	Fisher exact test, Chi square	McNemar test
	≥ 3	Pearson chi-square test	Cochran Q test
Binary outcome	—	Unconditional logistic regression	Conditional logistic regression
Continuous outcome	—	Linear regression	—

BOX 1-15   FISHER'S EXACT TEST

- When one or more of the expected, not the observed counts in a 2 × 2 table is small (< 2), the chi-square test cannot be used.
- The exact probability of finding the observed numbers which involves the Fisher's exact probability test is employed.

REFERENCES

1. Delgado-Rodriguez M, Lloroca J. *Bias. J Epidemiol Community Health.* 2004;58: 635–641.
2. Greenland S. Bias methods for sensitivity analysis of bases. *Int J Epidemiol.* 1996; 25:1107–1116.
3. Abrahamson JH. *Making Sense of Data.* 2nd ed. New York: Oxford University Press; 1994.
4. Garb JL. *Understanding Medical Research: A Practitioner's Guide.* Boston: Little, Brown, and Company; 2000.
5. Swinscow TDV, Campbell MJ. *Statistics at Square One.* 10th ed. Spain: BMJ Books; 2002.
6. Khan HA, Sempos CT. *Statistical Methods in Epidemiology.* New York: Oxford University Press; 1989.
7. Holcomb ZC. *Interpreting Basic Statistics.* 3rd ed. Los Angeles, CA: Pyrczak Publishing; 2002.
8. Kocher MS. Ultrasonographic screening for developmental dysplasia of the hip: an epidemiologic analysis (Part II). *Am J Orthop.* 2001;30:19–24.
9. Jekel JF, Katz L, Elmore JG. *Epidemiology, Biostatistics, and Preventive Medicine.* Philadelphia: Saunders; 2001.
10. Sackett DL, Richardson WS, Rosenberg W, Haynes RB. *Evidence-Based Medicine: How to Practice and Teach Evidence-Based Medicine.* 2nd ed. Edinburg: Churchill Livingstone; 2000.
11. Katz DL. *Clinical Epidemiology & Evidence-Based Medicine: Fundamental Principles of Clinical Reasoning & Research.* Thousand Oaks, CA: Sage; 2001.
12. Riegelman RK, Hirsch RP. *Studying a Test and Testing a Test.* 2nd ed. Boston: Little, Brown and Company; 1989.
13. Dawson-Saunders B, Trap RG. *Basic and Clinical Biostatistics.* 2nd ed. Norwalk, CT: Appleton & Lange; 1994.
14. Cronk BC. *How to Use SPSS. A Step-by-Step Guide to Analysis and Interpretation.* 3rd ed. Glendale, CA: Pyrczak Publishing; 2004.
15. Friedman GD. *Primer of Epidemiology.* 4th ed. New York: McGraw-Hill; 1994.
16. Altman DG. *Practical Statistics for Medical Research.* London: Chapman & Hall; 1991.
17. Armitage P, Berry G. *Statistical Methods in Medical Research.* 3rd ed. Oxford, U.K.: Blackwell Scientific Publishing; 1994.
18. Rosner B. *Fundamentals of Biostatistics.* 5th ed. Belmont, CA: Duxbury Press; 2000.
19. Freiman JA, Chalmers TC, Smith H, Kuebler RR. The importance of beta, the Type II error and sample size in the design and interpretation of the randomized clinical trial. *N Engl J Med.* 1978;299:690–694.
20. Fisher LD, van Belle G. *Biostatistics: A Methodology for Health Sciences.* 2nd ed. Hoboken, NJ: Wiley & Sons; 1993.
21. Colton T. *Statistics in Medicine.* New York: Little, Brown and Company; 1974.

22. Hollander M, Wolfe DA. *Nonparametric Statistical Methods.* 2nd ed. Hoboken, NJ: Wiley & Sons; 1998.

23. Conover WJ. *Practical Nonparametric Statistics.* Hoboken, NJ: Wiley & Sons; 1998.

24. Kleinbaum DG, Kupper LL, Muller KE. *Applied Regression Analysis and Other Multivariable Methods.* 2nd ed. Boston: PWS-KENT Publishing Company; 1998.

25. Meyers LS, Gamst G, Guarino AJ. *Applied Multivariate Research.* Thousand Oaks, CA: Sage Publications; 2006.

26. *STATA, Multivariate Statistics,* Release Version 10. College Station, Texas: STATA Press; 2007.

27. Rencher, AC. *Methods of Multivariate Analysis.* 2nd ed. New York: Wiley & Sons; 2002.

28. Hosmer DW, Lemeshow S. *Applied Logistic Regression Analysis.* 2nd ed. New York: Wilcy & Sons; 1989.

29. Kleinbaum DG, Klein M. *Logistic Regression.* 2nd ed. New York: Springer; 2002.

30. Kleinbaum DG, Klein M. *Survival Analysis.* 2nd ed. New York: Springer; 2005.

31. Cleves, MA, Gould WW, Gutierrez RG. *An Introduction to Survival Analysis Using STATA.* College Station, TX: STATA Press; 2004.

32. Kliein JP, Moeschberger ML. *Survival Analysis—Techniques for Censored and Truncated Data.* 2nd ed. New York: Springer; 2003.

33. Holmes, L, Chan W, Jiang Z, Du XL. Effectiveness of androgen deprivation therapy in prolonging survival of older men treated for logo-regional prostate cancer. *Prostate Cancer and Prostatic Diseases,* 2007. doi:10.1038/sj.pcan.4500973.

Chapter 2

Environmental Sciences in Public Health

Larry Holmes, Jr., and Jennifer Thompson

ENVIRONMENTAL SCIENCES CORE COMPETENCIES LEARNING OBJECTIVES

Environmental health sciences represent the study of environmental factors including biological, physical, and chemical factors that affect the health of a community.

PHCC.2.1.	Specify approaches for assessing, preventing, and controlling environmental hazards that pose risks to human health and safety.
PHCC.2.2.	Describe the direct and indirect human, ecological, and safety effects of major environmental and occupational agents.
PHCC.2.3.	Specify current environmental risk assessment methods.
PHCC.2.4.	Describe genetic, physiologic, and psychosocial factors that affect susceptibility to adverse health outcomes following exposure to environmental hazards.
PHCC.2.5.	Discuss various risk management and risk communication approaches in relation to issues of environmental justice and equity.
PHCC.2.6.	Explain the general mechanisms of toxicity in eliciting a toxic response to various environmental exposures.
PHCC.2.7.	Develop a testable model of environmental insult.
PHCC.2.8.	Describe federal and state regulatory programs, guidelines, and authorities that control environmental health issues.

PREVIEW

Public health originated from the initiative or effort to provide clean drinking water and avoid contaminated food. The *environmental* aspect of public health focused on these two aspects by controlling water and food safety, thus preventing diarrhea illnesses and mortality across human populations. With the modern environment, public health initiatives in this direction underwent a dramatic transition. Growing industries and the use of coal and fossil fuel resulted in increased levels of carbon dioxide emissions, increased global warming, and the contributions of environmental air pollutants and their interactions with oxygen at lower atmospheric levels, thus resulting in higher and higher ozone levels. In addition, the growth in industries and manufacturing has generated millions of tons of toxic heavy metals (manganese, nickel, chromium, cadmium), some of which are carcinogenic to humans, thus increasing human risk of cancer. Solid-waste generation and impaired disposal processes have increased during the past three decades as well as exposure to ionizing radiation.

The health effects of these environmental air, water, and soil pollutants contribute to the deteriorating health of the human population. The current role of the environmental sciences is to identify the environmental or toxic substances through risk assessment (and risk characterization), continue to evaluate the safety level of exposure of these substances, encourage the development of health policies to minimize their risk, and develop interventions to prevent exposure to these pollutants (air, water, heavy metals, biologic, solid hazardous wastes, ionizing radiation).

Environmental health is challenged with the explosive human population, given the degradation of water sources and increasing food scarcity as a result of deforestation and poor agricultural productivity. Thus, generating enough food to sustain the expanding human population remains the challenge of environmental public health in the nearest future. With the complexities of modern environment and emerging threats to the environment, environmental health sciences currently focuses on the impact of environmental conditions on human health, including disaster preparedness, epidemiology, occupational health, risk assessment, global warming, and climate changes. Environmental health sciences plays a role in identifying potentially harmful environmental exposures and examining health risk associated with natural, accidental, or terrorist emergencies and is challenged with developing diagnostic models to track the threats of global warming, climate changes, greenhouse effects, and environmental degradation.

This chapter presents the basic principles in risk assessment and environmental toxins as toxic substances and the impacts of those substances on human health or the health effects on the biological system. Risk characterization is the process by which the dose–response assessment and exposure assessments are integrated to predict risk to specific populations, whereas the final stage in the risk assessment process involves the prediction of the frequency and severity of effects in exposed populations. Also presented are the gender differences and psychosocial differentials in environmental health. Further, the role of governmental agencies in preventing the environmental factors that may affect human health is presented with specific focus on the federal regulatory body, the U.S. Environmental Protection Agency (EPA). In the same vein, mention is made of the Occupational Safety and Health Administration, which regulates safety in the workplace, and the Food and Drug Administration in the governmental effort to regulate the environment and protect the health of the population.

I.   **Environmental Sciences and Public Health**
   A. Historically, the role of environmental sciences in public health had been reducing and eliminating the incidence and prevalence of diseases caused and spread by contaminated water and food.
   B. Besides contaminated food and water, air contamination, radiation, pesticides, noise, motor vehicles, exposure to several occupational chemicals, and global warming present health hazards and are significant threats to the modern environment. [PHCC.2.2]
   C. Toxic pollutants [synthetic chemical waste, combustion products (air pollutants), chemical additives in food] act at the cellular level to initiate often-irreversible changes that can induce cellular damage and abnormal cellular proliferation.[1]
   D. Further examples are exposure to X-rays, organic chemicals, and heavy metals (such as mercury, manganese, chromium, cadmium), which can damage the cell or lead to neoplastic outcomes via uncontrolled cellular proliferation. [PHCC.2.2]
   E. The interaction of toxic substances in the environment may lead to:
      1. Mutation (point mutation, chromosomal aberrations, and change in chromosome numbers).[1,2]
      2. Birth defects (phocomelia, fetal alcohol syndrome).

3. Neoplastic disorders (cancers of various sites).

BOX 2-1   STEPS IN CARCINOGENESIS

- *Initiation* is the first step, and involves a change in the genetic material.
- Environmental carcinogens can bind to DNA nucleotides, thus forming DNA-carcinogenic adduct, leading to genetic damage and abnormal cellular proliferation.
- Second step involves a process by which the initiated cells are exposed to another group of agents termed *promoters*.
- Environmental agents play role in carcinogenesis as initiators, and promoters and both.

---

4. Chronic disease [cardiovascular disease, hypertension, stroke, asthma, chronic obstructive pulmonary disease (COPD)]. [PHCC.2.2]

F. *Environmental sciences as an applied core discipline of public health* presently deals with the identification of toxic pollutants or substances, their mechanisms of disease causation, and application of this knowledge and environmental policies to prevent and control environmental diseases, disabilities, injuries, and health-related events.

G. *Environmental health* deals with the burden of disease attributable to environmental factors.

1. Cause-and-effect relationships between water, air pollution, and human health have been well established.

2. Health consequences of other environmental factors and exposures, such as those resulting from climate change and chemicals in the environment, are a result of complex interactions between the environment and humans that are far less understood.

3. For some chemicals, such as endocrine-disrupting substances, the effects on humans are particularly difficult to unravel, but the impacts on wildlife have been substantial, with implications for human health.

4. Other chemicals in the environment, the disposal of wastes, and noise continue to generate concerns about their health effects on humans.[3]

H. Vulnerability and exposure, however, vary markedly between different groups and areas, with children and the elderly being particularly at risk.

I. Diseases associated with environmental factors have been well documented. Examples are allergies and asthma; neurotoxic effects of environmental contaminants; environmental factors influencing the onset of puberty; food and fertility; and cancer, heart disease, and obesity associated with risks correlated to environment, diet, and genetic factors.

1. Outdoor air pollution plays a role in the causation and aggravation of asthma and allergic responses, which are increasingly prevalent diseases, especially in children.

2. Much of the outdoor air penetrates indoors, and because people breathe both, an integrated approach to both outdoor and indoor air pollution is necessary.

3. Transport continues to be a significant contributor to health effects from accidents, air pollution, and noise.

Table 2-1	Types of Mutations
Mutation	**Description**
Point mutation	Involves a change at the molecular level within a gene
	Results from deletion or substitution of a base pair—impaired protein formation
	Most common type of mutation
Chromosomal aberration	Gross structural changes in the chromosome
	Caused by loss or addition of sizable pieces of a chromosome or reversing of chromosome part
	May result in lethal mutation
Change in chromosome number	Caused by nondisjunction or paired homologous chromosomes during meiosis

Table 2-2 Teratogens and Their Effects	
Teratogens	**Teratogenic Effect**
Microbes	
Toxoplasmosis	Central nervous system (CNS) abnormalities
Syphilis and herpes simplex type 2	Mental retardation, microcephaly, kidney and liver disorders, brain abnormalities
German measles	Congenital heart defect, deafness and hearing impairment, cataracts
Ionizing radiation	
X-rays	CNS disorders, microcephaly, visual disorders, and mental retardation
Drugs and chemicals	
Thalidomide	Phocomelia, or seal-limb, in which a hand or foot is attached directly to the torso without an arm or foot
Dioxin	Structural abnormalities and miscarriage
Dilantin	Heart malformations, cleft palate, mental retardation, microcephaly
Tobacco	Low birth weight, miscarriage, stillbirth
Valporic acid	Spina bifida
Tegison	Cardiovascular abnormalities, ear deformation, hydrocephaly, microcephaly
Accutane	Cardiovascular abnormalities, ear deformation, hydrocephaly, microcephaly
Anesthesia	Miscarriages and structural abnormalities
DES	Vagina cancer in girls and genital abnormalities in boys
Methyl mercury	Mental retardation, neuro-developmental disorders

II. **Health Hazards and Risk Assessment [PHCC.2.1, 2.3, 2.7]**

    A. Risk assessment involves an interdisciplinary approach among environmental epidemiology, environmental health policy, environmental health scientists, and governmental regulation. Risk assessment is loosely characterized as the use of the factual base to define the health effects of exposure of individuals or populations to hazardous materials and situations.[4] The four steps in risk assessment are: [PHCC.2.1, 2.3]

1. *Hazard identification:* seeks to address the question on the evidence of the agent and its potentials in developing a toxic effect in the exposed population.
2. *Exposure assessment:* attempts to identify those exposed with respect to medium (air, water, food), dosage, and the duration of exposure.
3. *Dose-response:* addresses the different doses (low, moderate, high) and their response in the exposed.
4. *Risk characterization:* addresses the predicted population health impact, given the exposure and the dose–response estimation in the exposed population.[4]

BOX 2-2   EXPOSURE ASSESSMENT

- A major aspect of the exposure assessment is to identify the exposure pathways.
- Also, all potential exposure pathways are carefully considered as well as contaminant releases, movement and fate in the environment and the exposed populations.

B. *Other characteristics*
1. *Risk* refers to undesirable consequence of a particular activity in relation to the likelihood that it may occur.
2. *Risk assessment* is an estimate of the likelihood of adverse effects that may result from exposure to certain health hazards (e.g., toxic substances in the environment).
3. *Risk management* decisions follow the identification and quantification of risk, which is determined by risk assessments.
4. During the regulatory process, *risk managers* may request that additional risk assessments be conducted to justify the risk management decisions.
5. Risk assessments may be conducted for individual chemicals or for complex mixtures of chemicals. In cases of complex mixtures, such as hazardous waste sites, the process of risk assessment itself becomes quite complex.

C. *Basic notions of risk assessment*
1. *Hazard* refers to the capability of a substance to cause an adverse effect.
2. *Risk* refers to the probability that the hazard will occur under specific exposure conditions.
3. *Risk assessment* refers to the process by which hazards, exposure, and risk are determined.
4. *Risk management* refers to the process of weighing policy alternatives and selecting the most appropriate regulatory action based on the results of risk assessment and social, economic, and political concerns.
   a. A risk is the chance that an adverse event will happen, multiplied by the extent of the effect.
   b. *Mathematically:* Risk $(R) = F \times E$, where F = frequency of the exposure and E = effect of exposure.
   c. Therefore, risk quantifies the product of the frequency and effect of an exposure (toxic substance).

Table 2-3   Steps in Risk Assessment Process

Step	Process	Description
I	Hazard identification	The health conditions associated with or caused by the pollutants
II	Exposure assessment	The amount of pollutant inhaled or ingested during a specific time period
		The number exposed
III	Dose–response assessment	The health conditions/problems at different exposure levels/doses
IV	Risk characterization	The extra risk (excess) of the health problems in the exposed population

D. *Basic steps in risk assessment* [PHCC.2.3, 2.7]
1. There are four basic steps in risk assessment, namely:
   a. *Hazard identification:* characterization of innate adverse toxic effects of agents.
   b. *Exposure assessment:* measurement or estimation of the intensity, frequency, and duration of human exposures to agents.

     c. *Dose–response assessment:* characterization of the relation between doses and incidences of adverse effects in exposed populations.

     d. *Risk characterization:* estimation of the incidence of health effects under the various conditions of human exposure.

2. Risk characterization depends totally on the first three steps of the risk process.

BOX 2-3   RISK CHARACTERIZATION

■ Risk characterization is the process in which the dose–response assessment and exposure assessments are integrated to predict risk to specific populations.

■ It is the final stage in the risk assessment process and involves the prediction of the frequency and severity of effects in exposed

---

E. *Hazard identification and dose–response assessment* [PHCC.2.1, 2.3, 2.7]

1. In this initial step, the potential for a xenobiotic to induce any type of toxic hazard is evaluated.

2. Information is gathered and analyzed in a weight-of-evidence approach.

3. The types of data usually consist of:

     a. Human epidemiology data.

     b. Animal bioassay data.

     c. Supporting data.

4. Based on these results, one or more toxic hazards may be identified:

     a. Cancer.

     b. Birth defects.

     c. Chronic toxicity.

     d. Neurotoxicity.

5. *Vignette:* Steps in cancer risk assessment involve:

     a. Qualitative evaluation of all epidemiology studies, animal bioassay data, and biological activity (e.g., mutagenicity).

       (1) The substance is classified as to carcinogenic risk to humans based on the weight of evidence.

(2) If the evidence is sufficient, the substance may be classified as a definite, probable, or possible human carcinogen.

b. Quantify the risk for those substances classified as definite or probable human carcinogens.

F. *Cancer classification schemes:* Initiation is the first step and involves a change in the genetic material. Environmental carcinogens can bind to DNA nucleotides, thus forming DNA-carcinogenic adducts, leading to genetic damage and abnormal cellular proliferation. The second step involves a process by which the initiated cells are exposed to another group of agents, termed *promoters*. Environmental agents play a role in carcinogenesis as initiators and promoters—and both.[1]

1. The two primary cancer classification schemes are:

   a. EPA.

   b. International Agency for Research on Cancer (IARC).

      (1) The EPA and IARC classification systems are quite similar.

      (2) The EPA's cancer assessment procedures have been used by several federal and state agencies. For example, the Agency for Toxic Substances and Disease Registry relies on the EPA's carcinogen assessments.

2. The EPA's cancer assessment procedures use several categories:

   a. The basis for sufficient human evidence is an epidemiology study that clearly demonstrates a causal relationship between exposure to the substance and cancer in humans.

   b. The data are determined to be limited evidence in humans if there are alternative explanations for the observed effect.

   c. The data are considered to be inadequate evidence in humans if no satisfactory epidemiology studies exist.

3. An increase in cancer in more than one species or strain of laboratory animals or in more than one experiment is considered sufficient evidence in animals.

4. Data from a single experiment can also be considered sufficient animal evidence if there is a high incidence or unusual type of tumor induced.

5. Normally, however, a carcinogenic response in only one species, strain, or study is considered as only limited evidence in animals.[5]

G. *Cancer slope:* The key risk assessment parameter derived from the EPA carcinogen risk assessment is the cancer slope factor.[5]
   1. This is a toxicity value that quantitatively defines the relationship between dose and response.
   2. The cancer slope factor is a plausible upper-bound estimate of the probability that an individual will develop cancer if exposed to a chemical for a lifetime of 70 years.
   3. The cancer slope factor is expressed as milligrams per kilograms per day (mg/kg/day).

H. The last step in risk assessment is to express the risk in terms of allowable exposure to a contaminated source.[5]

I. Risk is expressed in terms of the concentration of the substance in the environment where human contact occurs. For example, the unit risk in air is risk per milligram per cubic meter (risk/mg/m³), whereas the unit risk in drinking water is risk per milligram per liter (risk/mg/L). [PHCC.2.5]

J. For carcinogens, the media risk estimates are calculated by dividing cancer slope factors by 70 kg (average weight of man) and multiplying by 20 m³/day (average inhalation rate of an adult) or 2 L/day (average water consumption rate of an adult).

K. Exposure assessment involves exposed populations (general public or selected groups), types of substances (pharmaceuticals, occupational chemicals, or environmental pollutants), duration of exposure of a single substance or a mixture of substances (brief, intermittent, or protracted), and pathways and media (ingestion, inhalation, and dermal exposure).
   1. Exposure assessment is a key phase in the risk assessment process because without an exposure, even the most toxic chemical does not present a threat.
   2. All potential exposure pathways are carefully considered.
   3. Contaminant releases, their movement and fate in the environment, and the exposed populations are analyzed.

L. All possible types of exposure are considered in order to assess the toxicity and risk that might occur due to these variables:
   1. Physical environment.
   2. Potentially exposed populations.

M. The physical environment may include considerations of:
   1. Climate.
   2. Vegetation.

3. Soil type.
4. Groundwater.
5. Surface water.

N. Populations that may be exposed as the result of chemicals that migrate from the site of pollution are also considered.

O. Pollutants may:
1. Be transported away from the source.
2. Be physically, chemically, or biologically transformed.
3. Accumulate in various media.

P. *Exposure pathways* may include:
1. Groundwater.
2. Surface water.
3. Air.
4. Soil.
5. Food.
6. Breast milk.

Q. Because actual measurements of exposures are often not available, exposure models may be used. For example, in air quality studies, chemical emission and air dispersion models are used to predict the air concentrations to downwind residents. **[PHCC.2.7]**

R. *Risk characterization:* The final stage in the risk assessment process involves prediction of the frequency and severity of effects in exposed populations. **[PHCC.2.1, 2.3]**
1. Conclusions reached concerning hazard identification and exposure assessment are integrated to yield probabilities of effects likely to occur in humans exposed under similar conditions.
2. Because most risk assessments include major uncertainties, it is important that biological and statistical uncertainties are described in the risk characterization.
3. The assessment should identify which components of the risk assessment process involve the greatest degree of uncertainty.
4. In some complex risk assessments, such as for hazardous waste sites, the risk characterization must consider multiple chemical exposures and multiple exposure pathways.
5. Simultaneous exposures to several chemicals, each at a sub-threshold level, can often cause adverse effects by simple summation of injuries.

6. The assumption of dose additivity is most acceptable when substances induce the same toxic effect by the same mechanism.
7. When available, information on mechanisms of action and chemical interactions is considered and is useful in deriving more scientific risk assessments.
8. Individuals are often exposed to substances by more than one exposure pathway (e.g., drinking contaminated water, inhaling contaminated dust).
9. The total exposure will usually equal the sum of the exposures by all pathways.
10. *Higher exposure:* (a) living near an industrial complex, (b) living under a flight route, or (c) a child eating soil.
11. *More vulnerable:* (a) children, (b) pregnant women, (c) the elderly, and (d) COPD patients.

III. **Major Sources of Environmental Hazards and Their Health Impacts [PHCC.2.2, 2.4, 2.6]**
   A. Environmental hazards include, but are not limited to, air pollution, water pollution, solid waste, contaminated food, environmental factors, weaponized pathogens, and global warming (climate changes).
   B. *Outdoor air pollutants:* Major outdoor pollutants are particulate matter (PM), ozone, nitrogen oxide, carbon monoxide (CO), and sulfur dioxide.
   1. Power plants, factories, and vehicles spew out harmful gases and small particles that can penetrate deep into human lungs, causing health problems.
      a. In strong sunlight, oxides of nitrogen from vehicle exhaust fumes form ozone at ground level, which can trigger asthma attacks.
      b. Heavy metals and persistent organic pollutants are carried by winds, contaminating water and soil far from their origin.
      c. Industrial growth and rapid urbanization aggravate the problem, with the pressure felt most acutely in the megacities of the developing world.[6]
      d. Use of cleaner fuels and technologies, refined motor engines, and public transportation are crucial in ensuring that children breathe clean air.

2. *Scope of outdoor air pollution:* Worldwide, outdoor air pollution contributes to:
   a. Estimated 800,000 deaths per year.[7]
   b. Estimated 4.6 million healthy life-years lost per year.[7]
   c. 65% deaths and lost life-years in Asia alone.[7,8]
3. *Sources of outdoor air pollution:* May be quite different in rural and urban settings.
   a. Combustion of fossil fuels
      (1) Domestic heating.
      (2) Power generation.
      (3) Motor vehicles.
   b. Industrial processes
      (1) Cotton.
      (2) Rug-making.
   c. Waste incineration.
   d. Natural processes
      (1) Thunderstorms.
      (2) Volcanoes.
4. *Factors influencing outdoor air pollution*
   a. Climate: temperature, prevailing winds, and seasonal changes.
   b. Topography: hills and valleys and dominant vegetation.
   d. Cities.
   c. Surfaces.
5. *Particulate matter* refers to complex heterogeneous mixture of solid and liquid.
   a. *Sources:* (1) power plants and industry; (2) motor vehicles—domestic, coal burning; (3) natural sources (volcanoes, dust storms); and (4) small particles that form a surface for acid aerosol formation.
   b. Primary particles originating from combustion sources usually consist of a carbonaceous core with chemicals (such as sulfates, metals, and polycyclic aromatic hydrocarbons) adsorbed to their surfaces.[9]
   c. In addition, secondary particles are formed by chemical reactions in the atmosphere of primary particles with gases (such as nitric oxides, ozone, and sulfur oxides, which are strong oxidants), leading to formation of nitrates and ammonia.

  d. The specific composition and size distribution of PM varies by:

   (1) Region.

   (2) Time of year.

   (3) Time of day.

   (4) Weather conditions.

 6. PM and route of entry and deposition in human organs.

  a. Coarse particles (2.5–10 microns) deposited in the upper respiratory tract and large airways.[7]

  b. Fine particles (< 2.5 microns) may reach terminal bronchioles and alveoli.

  c. Particle size is the most important factor in determining where particles are deposited in the lung.

  d. Compared with large particles, fine particles can remain suspended in the atmosphere for longer periods and be transported over longer distances.

  e. Some studies suggest that fine particles have stronger respiratory effects in children than large particles.

 7. *Health effects of PM:* Deposition of fine particles in distal airways may cause:

  a. Acute respiratory morbidity (pneumonia, asthma).

  b. Increased mortality (from all causes).

  c. Decreased lung function in children.[9]

C. *Indoor air pollutants*

 1. *Sources:* Indoor air quality is influenced by: (a) concentrations of outdoor air pollutants, (b) indoor sources of pollution, and (c) characteristics of the building and the habits of the residents.[9]

 2. Indoor air pollution may arise from the use of open fires; unsafe fuels; or the combustion of biomass fuels, coal, and kerosene.

 3. Gas stoves or badly installed wood-burning units with poor ventilation and maintenance can increase the indoor levels of CO, nitrogen dioxide, and particles.

  a. Other pollutants not associated with fuel combustion include building materials such as asbestos and cement, wood preservatives, and others.

b. Volatile organic compounds (VOCs) may be released by various sources, including paints, glues, resins, polishing materials, perfumes, spray propellants, and cleaning agents.[3,9]
c. Formaldehyde is a component of some household products and can irritate the eyes, nose, and airways.

Table 2-4   Major Sources of Indoor Air Pollution

- Coal and biomass fuel can cause lung injury due to the inhalation of the ash particles.
- Suspended particulate matter increases the risk of acute respiratory infections.
- Carbon monoxide and other toxic gases may impair development and health.
- Second-hand tobacco smoke is a major concern.

---

4. *In summary:*
a. The indoor environment also reflects outdoor air quality and pollution.
b. Outdoor pollution primarily results from the combustion of fossil fuels by industrial plants and vehicles.
c. This releases CO, sulfur dioxide, PM, nitrogen oxides, hydrocarbons, and other pollutants.
d. The characteristics of emissions and solid-waste disposal may vary for each specific industry (e.g., smelting, paper production, refining, and others).

Table 2-5   Sources and Products of Combustion

Sources	Products
Gas stoves and appliances	Carbon monoxide
Wood and coal stoves	Nitrogen dioxide
Gas and propane engines	Sulfur dioxide
Fireplaces	Nitrogenated compounds
Tobacco smoke	Particulate matter
Candles and incense	
Mosquito coils	

   5. Chronic health conditions associated with indoor air pollutants.
      a. Decreased lung growth.
      b. Impaired pulmonary function.
      c. Increased susceptibility to chronic obstructive lung diseases, including asthma.

Table 2-6   Acute Health Consequences of Indoor Air Pollutants
■ Coughing, wheezing, chest tightness
■ Irritation of the mucous membranes (eyes, nose, throat)
■ Increased airway responsiveness to allergens
■ Increased incidence of acute respiratory illness
■ Pneumonia
■ Otitis media
■ Tracheobronchitis
■ Exacerbation of asthma

   D. *Solid fuels*
      1. Solid fuels comprise only 10 to 15% of fuel used.[10]
      2. Nearly one-half of the world's population uses solid fuels for heating homes and cooking.[7,8]
      3. Two billion people are exposed to PM and gases at levels up to 100 times higher than in ambient air.[7]
      4. Women and children are most exposed; levels may be 10 to 100 times above safety standards for ambient air.[7,8]
      5. Biomass (wood, agricultural produce, straw, and dung) produces a wide variety of liquids, suspended particles, gases, and mixtures.
      6. *Coal: Products and health impact*
         a. Benzene, formaldehyde, sulfur, heavy metals, and fluoride.
         b. Affect the most vulnerable populations: women of child-bearing age, infants, and children in the poorest circumstances.[6–9]
   E. *Carbon monoxide: Composition and physiochemical properties*
      1. CO is a colorless, odorless gas formed by incomplete burning of carbon-based fuels.

2. CO's affinity for hemoglobin (Hb) is 240 to 270 times greater than that of oxygen.[9]
    a. Decreases the capacity of Hb for carrying oxygen.
    b. Fetal Hb has a higher affinity for CO.
    c. CO causes a leftward shift of the oxyhemoglobin dissociation curve.
    d. Decreases oxygen delivery to tissues.
    e. Intoxication results in tissue hypoxia.

3. *Sources of carbon monoxide*
    a. *Gas, kerosene, wood stoves, and coal:* Incomplete oxidation during combustion in gas ranges and unvented gas or kerosene heaters may cause high concentrations of CO in indoor air.
    b. Worn or poorly adjusted and maintained combustion devices (e.g., boilers and furnaces) can be significant sources, especially if the fuel is of an unsuitable size, or if the system is blocked or leaking, such as chimneys and vents.
    c. Car, truck, or bus exhaust from attached garages, nearby roads, or parking areas can also be a source.
    d. CO is one of the components of tobacco smoke.[9]

Table 2-7   Ways to Prevent CO Poisoning

- Keep fuel-burning appliances in good working condition.
- Check heating systems, chimneys, and vents regularly.
- Never burn charcoal indoors.
- Never leave a car running in a garage.
- Install CO detectors.

F. *Second-hand smoke*
    1. Sources and composition of second-hand smoke
        a. Smoke released from cigarettes, cigars, and pipes is composed of more than 3,800 different substances.[7]
        b. Airborne PM is two to three times higher in homes of smokers.

    2.   Health impact of second-hand smoke
       a.   Respiratory tract illness and respiratory irritant symptoms.[10]
       b.   Asthma.
       c.   Middle ear effusions.
       d.   Prenatal complications and low birth weight.
       e.   Fire-related injuries.
       f.   Sudden infant death syndrome.
       g.   Cancer.
G. *Solvents and VOCs*
    1.   *Composition:* Organic chemicals are widely used as ingredients in household products including paints, varnishes, wax, cosmetics, degreasing agents, wood preservatives, aerosol sprays, cleansers, disinfectants, moth repellents, air fresheners, and hobby products (e.g., alkanes, aromatic hydrocarbons, alcohols, aldehydes, ketones).[9]
    2.   *Sources*
       a.   Solvents, fabric softeners, deodorizers, and cleaning products.
       b.   Paints, glues, resins, waxes, and polishing materials.
       c.   Spray propellants, dry cleaning fluids.
       d.   Pens and markers.
       e.   Binders and plasticizers.
       f.   Cosmetics, hair sprays, and perfumes.
       g.   Organic chemicals
          (1) All of these products can release organic compounds while they are being used, and, to some degree, when they are stored.
          (2) The average levels of several organic compounds in indoor air are two to five times higher than in outdoor air.[9]
          (3) During certain activities, such as paint stripping, and for several hours immediately afterward, levels may be 1,000 times higher than outdoor levels.
    3.   *Health impact of VOCs*
       a.   VOCs vary greatly in their health effects: some are highly toxic, whereas some have no known effects on health.
       b.   As with other pollutants, the extent and nature of the effects on health will depend on many factors, including level of exposure and duration of exposure.

    4. *Acute* health impacts of VOCs:
      a. Irritation of eyes and respiratory tract.
      b. Headache, dizziness, loss of coordination, nausea, visual disorders.
      c. Allergic reactions, including asthma and rhinitis.[9]
    5. *Chronic* health impacts of VOCs:
      a. Damage to liver, kidney, blood system, and the central nervous system (CNS).
      b. Cancer in humans.

H. *Biological pollutants*
    1. Animal dander, dust mites, molds, infectious agents, pollen.
    2. Sources
      a. Humidifiers and stagnant water.
      b. Water-damaged surfaces and materials.
      c. Water vapor from cooking and showering.
      d. Air-conditioning systems.
      e. Mattresses, upholstered furniture, and carpets.
    3. Dust mites, fungi, and bacteria require moisture to proliferate.
    4. Permeation of rain or groundwater into a building and condensation on cold interior surfaces can promote proliferation of microbes.
    5. Water vapor is produced by people and pets, cooking, and showering and requires sufficient air exchange to prevent moisture problems.
    6. Mattresses, upholstered furniture, and carpets are reservoirs for dust mites.
    7. Molds have been associated with two types of effects: (a) allergic reactions and (b) toxic effects. Toxic effects may be caused by inhalation of mycotoxins.
    8. Mold [PHCC.2.1]
      a. *Source:* Occurs in damp indoor spaces.[11]
      b. *Manifestations:* More common among individuals with atopic disease.
      c. Allergies and nonspecific symptoms are common, but infections are rare.
      d. *Mold-related diseases:*
        (1) Irritation of the airways and conjunctiva: Eye irritation, cough, and sore throat.
        (2) Headache.

(3) Difficulty in concentrating.

(4) Hypersensitivity reactions.

    (a) Asthma.

    (b) Allergic rhinitis.

(5) Infections

    (a) Thrush (candidiasis).

    (b) Systemic infections (immunosuppression).

(6) Acute toxicity: Linked to pulmonary hemorrhage in infants.

  e. Hypersensitivity to molds is immediate (type 1) and includes acute asthma, allergic rhinitis, and urticaria.

  f. Colonization associated with chronic asthma is rare and serious and includes allergic bronchopulmonary mycosis and allergic mycotic sinusitis.[12]

  g. Deep fungal infections are uncommon; serious, life-threatening diseases are not caused by common household molds.

    (1) The major exception is aspergillosis.

  h. Molds usually infect devitalized tissue or an immuno-compromised host.[13]

I. *Sick building syndrome* is assessed as follows:

  1. Discomfort is not related to specific illness.

  2. Effects appear to be linked to time spent inside the building.

  3. Cause of symptoms is unknown.[14]

  4. Most complaints are relieved soon after leaving the building (agent).

  5. *Manifestations:* Symptoms of identified illness attributed to airborne contaminants in the building.

  6. *Etiology*[14]

    a. Inadequate building design.

    b. Occupant activities.

    c. Remodeled buildings operating in a manner inconsistent with their original design.

    d. Inadequate ventilation.

    e. Inadequate maintenance.

    f. Chemical and biological contaminants.

  7. *Health impacts*

    a. Headache.

    b. Irritations of eyes, nose, or throat.[15]

   c. Dry cough.

   d. Dry or itchy skin.[16]

   e. Difficulty in concentrating.

   f. Fatigue.[16]

   g. Sensitivity to odors.

 J. Radon gas

  1. Composition

   a. Radon is a radioactive gas released from soil and rocks.[9]

   b. Geology of the area can predict levels in soil and water.

   c. Radon concentrations indoors depend on construction site and building materials.

   d. Radon is produced from the natural breakdown of thorium and uranium found in most rocks and soils. As it further breaks down, radon emits atomic particles.

   e. Radon is the second leading cause of lung cancer.[9,17–19]

  2. Source and mechanism of disease causation

   a. Highest levels occur in basements and on the ground floor.

   b. Radon is a radioactive gas that comes from the soil.

   c. These particles are in the air we breathe and can be deposited in the lungs.

   d. The energy associated with these particles can alter DNA, leading to an increased risk of lung cancer.

   e. Radon can enter a new house through cracks or pores in concrete flooring and walls or through openings in the foundations, floor–wall joints, or loose pipes.

  3. *Health impacts:* Exposure to radon gas is the second-leading cause of lung cancer (after smoking) in the United States.[17–20]

   a. About 14,000 people die each year from radon-related lung cancer.[20]

 K. *Ozone (O_3)*

  1. Structure, composition, and characteristics

   a. It is formed by photochemical reaction of VOCs, $NO_2 + O_2$.

   b. It peaks late afternoon.

   c. It is at its maximum level in hot, stagnant air.

   d. High concentrations increase asthma attacks in children.

   e. It is an important pollutant in many parts of the industrialized world.

f. It is rarely measured in developing countries, so there is less information about its role in those countries.

g. It is a naturally occurring form of oxygen that provides a protective layer shielding the Earth from harmful ultraviolet radiation.

h. It also occurs in the lower atmosphere.

i. It is the major component of urban smog and a potent respiratory irritant that can also synergistically enhance a child's reaction to other air pollutants and pollen.

j. It is a secondary air pollutant formed in the atmosphere from a chemical reaction between hydrocarbons and nitrogen oxides in the presence of heat and sunlight.

   (1) Ozone is a molecule composed of three atoms of oxygen.

   (2) The third oxygen atom can detach from the ozone molecule and reattach to molecules of other substances, thereby altering their chemical composition.

2. *Source:* Scientific evidence shows that at concentrations that do not exceed public health standards, ozone has little potential to remove indoor air contaminants; there is no approval for its use in occupied spaces.

Table 2-8 The Health Effect of Ozone

- When inhaled, ozone can damage the lungs.
- Relatively small amounts can cause chest pain, coughing, shortness of breath, and throat irritation.
- Ozone may also exacerbate chronic respiratory diseases such as asthma and compromise the ability of the body to fight respiratory infections.

Source: www.epa.gov/iaq/pubs/ozonegen.html.

L. *Chromium: Health impacts*

   1. *Acute poisoning*

      a. By ingestion: nausea, vomiting, hematemesis, acute renal failure.

      b. By inhalation: acute pneumonitis, runny nose, sneezing, nosebleeds.

      c. By skin contact: irritation, contact dermatitis, eczema.

      d. Allergies, which are the most common health effect of chromium, including

        (1) contact dermatitis and (2) eczema.

  2. *Reproductive toxicity*[9]

    a. Low birth weight.

    b. Birth defects.

    c. Disturbed spermatogenesis.

  3. *Cancer*

    a. Chromium is a human carcinogen and has been implicated in lung cancer.

M. *Cadmium*

  1. *Structure and composition*

    a. Pure cadmium ores are relatively rare; they are mostly contained in zinc and lead ores.

    b. Cadmium is widely used in industry: electroplating, production of steel, plastics, batteries, fertilizers, pigments, ceramics, and textiles.

  2. *Sources*

    a. *Inhalation*

      (1) Smoking and environmental tobacco smoke.

      (2) Industrial emission as in waste incineration.

    b. *Ingestion* (main route of exposure)

      (1) Food (internal organs of animals such as kidneys, tins of sardines, etc.).

      (2) Elevated levels in drinking water (impurities in the zinc of galvanized pipes and solders and metal fittings).

  3. *Health impacts*

    a. *Acute toxicity*

      (1) *Inhalation:* acute pneumonia.

      (2) *Ingestion:* nausea, vomiting, abdominal cramps, diarrhea, liver and/or kidney lesions.

      (3) Cadmium absorption has been reported to be as much as 3 to 8%. Several blood and dietary factors can influence the absorption of cadmium from the gastrointestinal tract. Dietary deficiencies of calcium or iron and diets low in protein content can enhance cadmium absorption.[9,21]

(a) Low blood ferritin content in women has been demonstrated to double the absorption of cadmium from the gastrointestinal tract. Zinc decreases the dietary absorption of cadmium.

b. *Chronic toxicity*

(1) *Inhalation:* implicated as a carcinogen in lung and prostate cancer.

(2) *Ingestion:* based on lesions of the tubular function of the kidney.

(3) Proteinuria (β_2-microglobulin).

(4) Decreased reabsorption of calcium and phosphorus leading to osteoporosis and osteomalacia, thus predisposing to bone and hip fractures.

(5) Hypertension.

(6) Impairment in B cell immune response.[9,21]

N. *Pesticides: Health impacts*

1. A number of epidemiologic studies have found a significant association between cancer and domestic exposure to pesticides.

2. Evidence is increasing but is still limited because of the methodological weaknesses of the research (e.g., retrospective and case-control designs that are weak in direct determination of risk).

3. The following malignancies have been associated with exposure to pesticides:

a. Brain tumor.

b. Acute lymphocytic leukemia.

c. Prostate cancer.

d. Non-Hodgkin's lymphoma.

4. Although pesticides are used specifically to kill pests, many of them have environmental impacts as well as toxic effects on humans. The environmental impact of their use includes resistance development, killing of beneficial species, and environmental contaminant.[2] The unintended contamination by pesticides may result in:

(a) Direct killing of organisms exposed to chemicals.

(b) Indirect killing via depletion of food or habitat.

(c) Groundwater contamination.

(d) Indirect contamination via food chains.

O. *Lead: Health impact*
  1. High blood lead level results in impaired intellectual ability in children.
  2. High affinity for nerve tissue and hence neurotoxicity— hyperirritability, impaired memory, convulsions, coma, and death at high levels.
  3. Interference with blood cell formation leading to anemia, as well as renal failure.[9]

IV. **Genetic, Physiologic, and Psychosocial Factors That Affect Susceptibility to Adverse Health Outcomes Following Exposure to Environmental Hazards [PHCC.2.4]**
  A. There are gender differences in environmental susceptibilities, implying the assessment of differences and similarities between men and women with respect to susceptibility to environmental factors in health.
    1. This has been shown in areas of research such as work on environmental estrogens and multiple chemical exposures. Gender differences in response to toxic substances, allergens, and autoimmune and other immune responses to environmental factors have been reported.[22] Infectious agents, emerging infections, repeated exposure to childhood infections, and differential exposures among child care workers (most of whom are women) have been reported to have differential health outcomes between populations of men and women.
  B. Ultraviolet radiation presents with varying exposure experience; thus men are more likely to work outdoors, whereas women are more likely to sunbathe. Dietary and environmental estrogens as variables of the hormonal cycle and changes in dietary behavior increase exposure to phytoestrogens.
    1. Detoxifying the body, such as chelation agents to bind and remove a toxicant, particularly in the detoxifying process, makes once-stored agents more bioavailable.
    2. Because men and women spend different amounts of time outside, the effect of ozone on health presents with gender differentials.
    3. Race, ethnicity, and culture may play a role in establishing differential exposures between men and women of a given

subpopulation or between women of different racial, ethnic, or cultural groups.[22]

4. Psychosocial conditions and susceptibility to environmental disease are also factors. [PHCC.2.4] Disadvantaged communities face greater likelihood of exposure to ambient hazards.[22]

   a. Ethnicity is highly correlated with residential location, with minorities and whites often living segregated from one another. Differential residential location comes with differential exposure to health risks.

   b. Disadvantaged communities encounter greater exposure to environmental toxicants such as air pollution, pesticides, and lead.

5. The exposure–disease paradigm has long suggested that differential "vulnerability" may modify the effects of toxicants on biological systems.

6. Psychosocial stress may be the vulnerability factor that links social conditions with environmental hazards.

7. Psychosocial stress can lead to acute and chronic changes in the functioning of body systems (e.g., immune) and also lead directly to illness.

8. Both individual and community stressors interrelate and correlate positively.

9. When community stressors and pollution sources outweigh neighborhood resources, levels of community stress manifest or increase.

   a. Community stress is a state of ecologic vulnerability that may translate into individual stressors, which in turn may lead to individual stress.

   b. Individual stress may then make individuals more vulnerable to illness when they are exposed to environmental hazards.

10. The exposure–disease paradigm is a well-known model that shows how environmental toxicants might cause disease.[23,24]

11. It is a continuum that includes the emission of a contaminant from a source through human exposure to the occurrence of a health effect.

12. Studies have reported that segregation is associated with numerous outcomes, including infant mortality,[25] adult

mortality,[26] tuberculosis, homicide,[27] teenage childbearing, exposure to tobacco and alcohol advertising,[28] and increased exposure to air pollution.[29]

13. Structural factors are constraints that shape how new conditions emerge, such as "salutogens" factors that promote health and those that serve as risks to health may be especially pertinent to environmental health disparities and include the local and national economy, neighborhood physical conditions, land use patterns, and health infrastructure.

V. **Mechanism of Disease Causation with Environmental Pollutants and Toxins [PHCC.2.6]**

A. *Asbestos:* Fibers inhaled past the mucociliary escalator accumulate primarily at alveolar duct bifurcations, thus explaining the pattern of developing asbestosis as the lesions begin near the bronchioles and spread peripherally along the alveolar ducts over time, demonstrating a localized dose response. Inhaled fibers that deposit on the type I alveolar epithelial surfaces are rapidly translocated by these cells to the interstitial vascular and lymphatic spaces from where they can reach the pleura and other anatomic compartments.

B. *Cyanide:* Binding to cytochrome oxide within the mitochondria and ferric iron (Fe^{3+}) complex leads to the blocking of oxidative phosphorylation, resulting in impaired oxygen extraction and utilization by the mitochondria leading to hypoxia—the abrupt cessation of cellular respiration.[9]

C. *Polychlorinated biphenyls (PCBs)*

1. PCBs and related halogenated aromatics as inducers of drug-metabolizing enzymes and the activity of individual compounds are remarkably dependent on structure.

2. PCBs typically cause thymic atrophy (a wasting syndrome), immunotoxic responses, reproductive problems, porphyria, and related liver damage.

3. In PCB-exposed animals, these effects are preceded by the induction of numerous enzymes, including the hepatic and extrahepatic drug-metabolizing enzymes. PCBs exhibit a wide range of toxic effects.

4. These effects may vary depending on the specific PCB. Similar to dioxin, toxicity of coplanar PCBs and mono-ortho-PCBs are

thought to be primarily mediated via binding to an aryl hydro-carbon receptor (AhR).[30] Because AhR is a transcription factor, abnormal activation may disrupt cell function by altering the transcription of genes.

5. The concept of toxic equivalency factors is based on the ability of a PCB to activate AhR. However, not all effects may be mediated by the AhR receptor. For example, di-ortho-substituted non-coplanar PCBs interfere with intracellular signal transduction dependent on calcium; this may lead to neurotoxicity.[31] Ortho-PCBs may disrupt thyroid hormone transport by binding to transthyretin.[32]

D. *Dioxin—2,3,7,8-tetrachlorodibenzo-p-dioxin (TCDD)*

1. TCDD's initial action is mediated through binding to the receptor, followed by processing, translocation into the nucleus, and eventual activation of a variety of genes for transcriptional processing. Therefore, it is unlikely that TCDD directly binds with the glucose transporter protein to cause inhibition of its transporting capability.

2. Lipoprotein lipase (LPL) is important in the process of triglyceride storage in adipose tissue. Depression of LPL activity in adipose tissue is associated with TCDD-induced wasting syndrome and may have a role in the associated serum hyperlipidemia produced by TCDD.[33]

E. *Insecticides:* Most modern insecticides are neurotoxicants and neuroexcitants.

1. Those that affect cholinesterase (organophosphates and carbamates) cause an increase in the postsynaptic concentrations of acetylcholine, which interacts with its receptor to increase neural activities.

2. Nicotine derivatives act as imitators of acetylcholine to stimulate its receptor as well. There are two large classes of insecticides that affect either the sodium channels [pynethnoids and 1,1,1-trichloro-2,2-bis(pchlorophenyl) ethane, on DDT] or the gamma-aminobuytric acid receptors (e.g., cyclodienes).

3. In all cases, acutely affected animals show a typical pattern of hyperexcitation and, at high doses, paralysis and death. Depletion of glycogen storage is a frequently observed result, indicating that a stimulation of glycogenolytic and glycolytic activities accompanies hyperexcitation.

4. A limited number of insecticides (e.g., chlordimeform and amitraz) are known to act as pseudoagonists to receptors for biogenic amines or to increase their concentrations by interfering with their metabolism and/or reuptake.

F. *Lead*

1. Once absorbed within the body, lead can interfere with body functions that rely heavily upon the activity of calcium.

2. Lead interferes with the production of the oxygen-carrying component of blood called hemoglobin, leading to a decreased ability of red blood cells to carry oxygen.

3. Lead has also been documented to damage and modify the function of kidneys, bone, nervous system, circulatory system, and gastrointestinal tract.

4. Lead poisoning results from the interaction of the metal with biological electron-donor groups, such as the sulfhydryl groups, which interferes with a multitude of enzymatic processes. Lead also interacts with essential cations, particularly calcium, iron, and zinc; it interferes with the sodium-potassium-adenosine triphosphate (Na^+/K^+-ATP) pump; and it alters cellular and mitochondrial membranes, thereby increasing cellular fragility. Additionally, lead inhibits pyrimidine-5′-nucleotidase and alters other nucleotide functions.[34]

5. Lead interferes with many enzyme systems of the body, thereby affecting the function of virtually every organ. Clinical manifestations of lead toxicity include symptoms referable to the CNS, the peripheral nervous system, the hematopoietic system, the renal system, and the gastrointestinal system. Children exposed to lead may experience devastating consequences because of the effects of lead on the developing brain.

G. *Mercury:* Precise mechanism is unknown, but it has been postulated to induce oxidative stress. Mitochondrial damage from oxidative stress has been observed to be the earliest sign of neurotoxicity with methylmercury.

1. A study in neural tissue indicates the electron transport chain appears to be the site where free radicals are generated, leading to oxidative damage induced by methylmercury.

2. Mercury can cause biochemical damage to tissues and genes through diverse mechanisms, such as interrupting intracellular calcium homeostasis, disrupting membrane potential, altering protein synthesis, and interrupting excitatory amino acid pathways in the CNS.[35] Mitochondrial damage, lipid peroxidation, microtubule destruction,[36] and the neurotoxic accumulation of serotonin, aspartate, and glutamate are all mechanisms of methylmercury neurotoxicity.[35]

H. *Cadmium:* Exposure of primary suspension cultures of isolated rat hepatocytes to cadmium has been shown to result in a dose-dependent reduction in the synthesis of cellular proteins.[37]

1. Changes in the kidney due to cadmium toxicosis have been well established. Chronic exposure to cadmium by the oral or inhalation routes has produced proximal tubule cell damage, proteinuria (mainly low molecular weight proteins, such as β_2-microglobulin), glycosuria, amino aciduria, polyuria, decreased absorption of phosphate, and enzymuria in humans and in a number of laboratory animal species.

2. Cadmium has been shown to perturb lipid composition and enhance lipid peroxidation. Depletion of antioxidant enzymes, specifically glutathione peroxidase and superoxide dismutase, has been proposed as the mechanism of cadmium's cardiotoxic effects, but subsequent studies showed that cardiotoxic mechanisms other than peroxidation are also present.[38]

3. Cadmium has been shown to alter zinc, iron, and copper metabolism[39] as well as selenium.[38]

VI. **Environmental Protection Agency and Regulatory Entities [PHCC.2.8]**

A. The Code of Federal Regulations (CFR) Title 40 is the section of the CFR that deals with protection of the environment and has a distinct mission of protecting human health and the environment through the EPA.

B. Primarily, the EPA develops and enforces regulations that embrace many environmental categories, from acid rain reduction to wetlands restoration. For example, PCBs are primarily employed as cooling liquids in electrical transformers and capacitors. The EPA estimates that 91% of all Americans have detectable levels of PCBs in their fatty tissues. The EPA offices include:

1. Office of Air and Radiation.
2. Office of Prevention, Pesticides, and Toxic Substances.
3. Office of Solid Waste and Emergency Response.
4. Office of Water.

Table 2-9   Offices and Regulations of Environmental Protection Agencies

Offices	Regulation—Law	Subsections and Guidelines
Office of Air and Radiation (OAR)	The Clean Air Act (CAA) is a statute written by Congress that gives the EPA the authority to establish regulations, policy, and guidance to protect air quality.	The CAA requires the EPA to regulate emissions of toxic air pollutants from a published list of industrial sources referred to as "source categories."
Office of Prevention, Pesticides, and Toxic Substances (OPPTS)	OPPTS plays an important role in protecting public health and the environment from potential risk of pesticides and toxic chemicals for now and for generations to come. Promotes pollution prevention through innovative partnerships and collaboration.	Office of Pesticide Programs (OPP)* Office of Pollution Prevention and Toxics (OPPT)‡ Office of Science Coordination and Policy (OSCP)§
Office of Solid Waste and Emergency Response (OSWER)	The Resource Conservation and Recovery Act (RCRA) is the public law that creates the framework for the proper management of hazardous and nonhazardous solid waste.	RCRA is the primary U.S. law governing the disposal of solid and hazardous waste. Congress passed RCRA on October 21, 1976, to address the increasing problems the nation faced from our growing volume of municipal and industrial waste.#

		Subsections and
Offices	**Regulation—Law**	**Guidelines**
Office of Water (OW)	Safe Drinking Water Act Amendments of 1996	The Safe Drinking Water Act Amendments of 1996 (PL 104-182) established a new charter for the nation's public water systems and the EPA in protecting the safety of drinking water.

Table 2-9   Offices and Regulations of Environmental Protection Agencies *(continued)*

*OPP promotes the use of safer chemicals, processes, and technologies; promotes life-cycle management of environmental problems such as asbestos; advances pollution prevention through voluntary action by industry.

†Through the high-production volume challenge program, for example, OPPT is working voluntarily with industry and others to make basic hazard data available to the public on more than 2,200 chemicals used in high volume in the United States, and to identify and evaluate chemicals of particular concern to children's health.

§OSCP provides coordination, leadership, and peer review on science and science policy within OPPTS.

#RCRA provides, in broad terms, the general guidelines for the waste management program envisioned by Congress. It includes a congressional mandate directing the EPA to develop a comprehensive set of regulations to implement the law. These regulations, or rulemakings, issued by the EPA, translate the general mandate of the law into a set of requirements for the agency and the regulated community. RCRA, which amended the Solid Waste Disposal Act of 1965, set national goals for:

• Protecting human health and the environment from the potential hazards of waste disposal.

• Conserving energy and natural resources.

• Reducing the amount of waste generated.

• Ensuring that wastes are managed in an environmentally sound manner.

C. The *Safe Drinking Water Act* (SDWA) was originally passed by Congress in 1974 to protect public health by regulating the nation's public drinking water supply. The law was amended in 1986 and 1996 and requires many actions to protect drinking water and its sources: rivers, lakes, reservoirs, springs, and groundwater wells. The 1996 amendment included, among other things, new prevention approaches, improved consumer information, changes to improve the regulatory program, and funding for state and local water systems. (SDWA does not regulate private wells that serve fewer than 25 individuals.) SDWA authorizes the EPA to set national health-based standards for drinking water to protect against both naturally occurring and man-made contaminants that may be found in drinking water.

VII. **EPA, Environmental Justice, and Public Health [PHCC.2.5]**
   A. The notion of environmental justice (EJ) is essential in addressing psychosocial, gender, and other socio-demographic differentials in susceptibility to environmental factors in disease and health of the population.
   B. *Environmental justice movement* refers to the community's action to oppose racial and economic inequities in the burden of environmental health hazards. This movement embraces the traditions of labor, civil rights, economic justice, environmental, and antiwar organizations. The objective of this movement is to mobilize the community to improve living and working conditions and quality of life in communities that have high disease rates and poor access to medical care and health-promoting services.[40,41] Retrospective data have indicated that the EJ movement may play an important role in public health improvement through its effects on the environment. The evidence from the epidemiologic transition validates these historical data. As clearly observed, most of the decline of mortality from infectious diseases between the mid-19th and mid-20th centuries occurred before introduction of effective medical interventions as a function of improved nutrition, sanitation, housing, working conditions, and reduced crowding.
   C. The EPA describes *environmental justice* as the fair treatment for people of all races, cultures, and incomes, regarding the development of environmental laws, regulations, and policies. Over the last decade, attention to the impact of environmental pollution on particular segments of our society has been steadily growing. Disparities in the adverse effect of the environment on health have been observed. This observation that minority populations and/or low-income populations bear a disproportionate amount of adverse health and environmental effects led President Bill Clinton to issue Executive Order 12898 in 1994, focusing federal agency attention on these issues. The EPA responded by developing the *Environmental Justice Strategy,* which focuses on the agency's efforts to address these concerns.

REFERENCES

1. Nasca PC, Pastides H. *Fundamentals of Cancer Epidemiology*. Frederick, MD: Aspen Publishers; 2001.
2. Nadakaavukaren A. *Our Global Environment: A Health Perspective*. 5th ed. Long Grove, IL: Waveland Press; 2000.
3. U.S. Environmental Protection Agency. "Municipal Solid Waste Basic Facts." www.epa.gov/epaoswer/non-hw/muncpl/facts.htm. Accessed March 12, 2008.
4. National Research Council, National Academy of Sciences. *Risk Assessment in the Federal Government: Managing the Process*. Washington, DC: National Academy Press; 1983.
5. U.S. Environmental Protection Agency. *Guidelines for Carcinogen Risk Assessment* (2005). http://cfpub.epa.gov/ncea/cfm/recordisplay.cfm?deid=116283. Accessed February 29, 2008.
6. Molina LT. Megacities and atmospheric pollution. *J Air Waste Manag Assoc*. 2004; 54:644.
7. World Health Organization. *Development of WHO Guidelines for Indoor Air Quality*. Report on a working Group Meeting. Bonn, Germany, October 23–24, 2006.
8. Suk WA, Ruchirawat KM, Balakrishnan K, et al. Environmental Threats to Children's Health in Southeast Asia and the Western Pacific. *Environmental Health Perspectives*. 2003;111:1340–1347.
9. U.S. Environmental Protection Agency. *Air and Radiation, Air Pollution*. http://www.epa.gov/air/airpollutants.html. Accessed November 28, 2008.
10. Pilkington PA, Gray S, Gilmore AB. Health impacts of second hand smoke (SHS) amongst a highly exposed workforce: survey of London casino workers. *BMC Public Health*. 2007;7:257. doi 10.1186/1471-2458-7-257.
11. U.S. Environmental Protection Agency. *Indoor Air Pollution: An Introduction for Health Professionals*. www.epa.gov. Accessed November 12, 2007.
12. U.S. Department of Health and Human Services. Centers for Disease Control and Prevention. *Environmental Hazards and Health Effects: Mold*. http://cdc.gov/mold/ & http://www.cdc.gov/nceh/.
13. U.S. Department of Health and Human Services. Centers for Disease Control and Prevention. *Environmental Health*. http://www.cdc.gov/Environmental/. Accessed December 3, 2007.
14. Marmot AF, Eley J, Stafford M, et al. Building health: an epidemiological study of "sick building syndrome" in the Whitehall II study. *Occup Environ Med*. 2006;63:283–289.
15. Assoulin-Daya Y, Leong A, Shoenfeld Y, et al. Studies of sick building syndrome. IV. Mycotoxicosis. *J Asthma*. 2002;39:191–201.
16. Apte MG, Fisk WJ, Daisey JM. Associations between indoor CO_2 concentrations and sick building syndrome symptoms in U.S. office buildings: an analysis of the 1994-1996 BASE study data. *Indoor Air*. 2000;10:246–257.
17. Field RW, Steck DJ, Smith BJ, et al. Residential radon gas exposure and lung cancer: The Iowa Radon Lung Cancer Study. *Am J Epidemiol*. 2000;151:1091–1102.

18. Lubin JH, Boice JD Jr. Lung cancer risk from residential radon: meta-analysis of eight epidemiologic studies. *J Natl Cancer Inst.* 1997;89:49–57.

19. Lubin JH. Indoor radon and the risk of lung cancer. *Radiat Res.* 1999;151: 105–107.

20. U.S. Environmental Protection Agency. *Health Effects of Radon.* http://www.epa. gov/radiation/docs/assessment/402-r-03-003.pdf.

21. U.S. Environmental Protection Agency. *Toxic Effect of Cadmium.* http://www. atsdr.cdc.gov/toxprofiles/tp5.pdf. Accessed December 24, 2007.

22. Sexton K, Olden K, Johnson BL. "Environmental justice": The central role of research in establishing a credible scientific foundation for informed decision making. *Toxicol Ind Health.* 1993;9:685–727.

23. Lioy PJ. Measurement methods for human exposure analysis. *Environ Health Perspect.* 1995;103(3):35–44.

24. Letz R, Ryan PB, Spengler JD. Estimating personal exposures to respirable particles. *Environ Monit Assess.* 1984;4:351–359.

25. Racial/Ethnic Disparities in Infant Mortality—United States, 1995–2002. *MMWR.* 2005, June 10;54(22):553–556.

26. Jackson SA, Anderson RT, Johnson NJ, Sorlie PD. The relation of residential segregation to all-cause mortality: A study in black and white. *Am J Public Health.* 2000;90:615–617.

27. Peterson RD, Krivo LJ. Racial segregation, the concentration of disadvantage, and black and white homicide victimization. *Sociol Forum.* 1999;14:465–493.

28. Alaniz ML. Alcohol availability and targeted advertising in racial/ethnic minority communities. *Alcohol Health Res World.* 1998;22:286–289.

29. Lopez R. Segregation and black/white differences in exposure to air toxics in 1990. *Environ Health Perspect.* 2002;110(suppl 2):289–295.

30. Safe S, Bandiera S, Sawyer T, et al. PCBs: Structure-function relationships and mechanism of action. *Environ Health Perspect.* 1985;60:47–56.

31. Chauhan KR, Kodavanti PR, McKinney JD. Assessing the role of ortho-substitution on polychlorinated biphenyl binding to transthyretin, a thyroxine transport protein. *Toxicol Appl Pharmacol.* 2000;162(1):10–21.

32. Woods SL, Trobaugh DJ. Polychlorinated biphenyl reductive dechlorination by vitamin B12s: thermodynamics and regiospecificity. *Environ Sci Technol.* 1999; 33:857–863.

33. Oslen H, Enan E, Matsumura F. 2,3,7,8-tetrachlorodibenzo-*p*-dioxin mechanism of action to reduce lipoprotein lipase activity in the 3T3-L1 preadipocyte cell line. *J Biochem Toxicol.* 1998;2:29–39.

34. *Mechanism of Lead.* //www.emedicine.com/MED/topic1269.htm. Accessed April 15, 2008.

35. Yee S, Choi BH. Oxidative stress in neurotoxic effects of methylmercury poisoning. *Neurotoxicology.* 1996;17:17–26.

36. National Research Council. *Toxicological Effects of Methylmercury.* Washington, DC: National Academy Press; 2000:54–55.

37. Din WS, Frazier JM. Protective effect of metallothionein on cadmium toxicity in isolated rat hepatocytes. *Biochem J.* 1985;230:395–402.

38. Jamall IS, Naik M, Sprowls JJ, et al. A comparison of the effects of dietary cadmium on heart and kidney oxidant enzymes: Evidence for the greater vulnerability of the heart to cadmium toxicity. *J Appl Toxicol.* 1989;9:339–345.

39. Petering HG, Choudhury H, Stemmer KL. Some effects of oral ingestion of cadmium on zinc, copper and iron metabolism. *Environ Health Perspect.* 1979;28:97–106.

40. Lee C. Environmental justice: Building a unified vision of health and the environment. *Environ Health Perspect.* 2002;110(suppl 2):141–144.

41. Krieger N. Embodying inequality: A review of concepts, measures, and methods for studying health consequences of discrimination. *Int J Health Serv.* 1999;29:295–352.

Chapter 3

Principles and Methods of Epidemiology

Larry Holmes, Jr.

EPIDEMIOLOGY CORE COMPETENCIES LEARNING OBJECTIVES

Epidemiology is the study of patterns of disease and injury in human populations and the application of this study to the control of health problems.

PHCC.3.1.	Explain the importance of epidemiology for informing scientific, ethical, economic, and political discussion of health issues.
PHCC.3.2.	Describe a public health problem in terms of magnitude, person, time, and place.
PHCC.3.3.	Apply the basic terminology and definitions of epidemiology.
PHCC.3.4.	Identify key sources of data for epidemiologic purposes.
PHCC.3.5.	Calculate basic epidemiology measures.
PHCC.3.6.	Evaluate the strengths and limitations of epidemiologic reports.
PHCC.3.7.	Draw appropriate inferences from epidemiologic data.
PHCC.3.8.	Communicate epidemiologic information to lay and professional audiences.
PHCC.3.9.	Comprehend basic ethical and legal principles pertaining to the collection, maintenance, use, and dissemination of epidemiologic data.
PHCC.3.10.	Identify the principles and limitations of public health screening programs.

PREVIEW

Epidemiology is simply a population-oriented discipline that quantifies, locates, and determines causes and mechanisms of health-related states or events and applies this knowledge to prevention and control of health-related events in specified populations. Epidemiology has been traditionally defined as the study of the distribution and determinants of health-related events in the human population and the application of this knowledge to disease, disability, and injury control and prevention. As a basic science of public health, epidemiology is involved in the assessment and monitoring of health status at the population level and the application of these results in disease prevention and control.[1] Specifically, epidemiology deals with (1) measurement of disease occurrence and frequency in the population; (2) identification of when, where, and within which population subgroups health-related events are more or less likely to occur; (3) determining the causes at the population level; (4) determining the mechanisms of causation, natural history, and the clinical course of the health-related events; and (5) application of the results to the prevention and control of disease and health-related events.[1,2]

This chapter presents the definition and role of epidemiology in public health in relation to the core functions of public health, mainly descriptive epidemiology which refers to (1) place, (2) person, and (3) time. Measures of disease frequency and occurrence and types of epidemiologic designs are also discussed: (1) ecologic, (2) cross-sectional, (3) case-control, (4) cohort, and (5) experimental (clinical trial). Each epidemiologic design is followed by an in-depth review of the study description, measures of association or point estimate, and advantages and limitations of each design. Both internal and external validity of epidemiologic studies are reviewed, with emphasis on confounding, bias as systematic error, random error, effect measure modifier or interaction, and epidemiologic causal inference. Also, the importance of epidemiology in informing scientific, ethical, economic, and political discussion in health issues is presented as well as the ethical and legal responsibilities of epidemiology in study designs, data collection, and results dissemination. Further, the basic principles of disease screening, advantages, limitations, and related biases are highlighted. Finally, the role of epidemiology in health policy development is addressed with the notion that health policy development requires objective information regarding risk factors in order to design and implement interventions that are data based.

I. **Definition of Epidemiology [PHCC.3.1, 3.3]**
   A. Basic science of human public health that deals with the *distribution, determinants,* and *prevention* of disease, disabilities, and injuries in human populations.
      1. Because public health is incomplete without animal health, the definition of epidemiology transcends human population and embraces animal populations, which is the focus of veterinary public health.
   B. Study of the distribution and determinants of health-related states or events in *specified populations,* and the *application* of this study to the control of health problems.
      1. *Distribution* implies the frequency (number, percentage, prevalence, rates, ratio, risk) and pattern (time, place, person) of health events in a population.
      2. *Determinants* imply the causes, variables, and factors influencing the health-related events with respect to their occurrences.
      3. *Specified population* implies the collective health of the population/people in a community setting in contrast to clinical medicine, which is concerned with the health of an individual patient.
      4. *Application:* Whereas the primary role of epidemiology is not to control or prevent health-related events, it provides data for public health action in controlling and preventing diseases, disabilities, and injuries.[1]
   C. Epidemiology, which originates from *epidemic,* comes from the Greek word *epi* (upon) and *demos* (people). An epidemic implies the occurrence of disease, disability, and injury beyond the usual or the expected (out of proportion).
      1. *Vignette:* A city of Notown, Texas, with a population of 246,000, normally has an incidence of Shigellosis of 5.0 / 1,000 during the summer months. In summer 2006, the incidence was 125.0 / 1,000.
      2. The occurrence of new cases (incidence) in 2006 clearly illustrates an epidemic of Shigellosis in Notown, Texas.

Table 3-1 Descriptive and Analytic Epidemiology	
Descriptive Epidemiology	**Analytic Epidemiology**
Disease occurrence data with respect to time, place, and person	Disease causes data with respect to the rate of occurrence, the differences in rates, and why the differences occurred
Provides information on what, who, when, and where	Provides information on why and how

II. Role of Epidemiology in Public Health [PHCC.3.1, 3.3]

    A. Epidemiology focuses on the assessment of disease, disabilities, and injuries at the population level.

    B. The knowledge gained from epidemiology is used to design intervention in order to prevent and control diseases, disabilities, and injuries at the population level.

    C. Epidemiology is the tool for public health to use in its mission of disease control and health promotion. Epidemiology in public health is, therefore, an applied science providing analytic input to the understanding of health and health-related issues.

    D. The focus of public health is to control and prevent disease, as well as promote health, whereas that of epidemiology is to assess the health condition involving the assessment of diseases, disabilities, and injuries, as well as health-related states.[3]

        1. *Vignette:* The Delaware State Department of Human Services is responding to increasing cases of childhood leukemia and lymphoma (hematological tumors). The chief epidemiologist proposes to examine the determinants of these tumors. The epidemiologist's role in this context is that of disease assessment, not control and prevention or health promotion. If the director of the department proposes to address the determinants of these hematological tumors by starting an intervention to eliminate environmental carcinogens, this approach illustrates the health promotion role of public health.

Table 3-2   The Focus of Epidemiology and Public Health*

Epidemiology (Core Focus)	Public Health (Core Focus)
Assessment of diseases, disabilities, and injuries (health phenomena)	Control and prevention of diseases, disabilities, and injuries, as well as health promotion
Distribution (frequency) and determinants (risk and protective factors)	Intervention, design, and implementation to address disease, disabilities, and injuries' risk, and protective factors

* The primary focus of epidemiology is not to control and prevent diseases, disabilities, and promote population health.[3] This is the primary function/role of public health.

III. History and Modern Concept of Epidemiology

Table 3-3   History of Modern Epidemiology

Person	Contribution to Disease Causation	Time (Period)
Hippocrates	Environmental and host factors in the development of a disease	Circa 400 B.C.
John Graunt— first epidemiologist, statistician, and demographer	Quantification of patterns of birth, death, and disease occurrence; bills of fertility, morbidity, and mortality on weekly count of death in London	1662
James Lind— surgeon with interest in epidemiology	Conducted one of the earliest experimental investigations on the treatment of scurvy; attributed causes of scurvy to moist air and diet	1747
William Farr— trained physician and self-taught mathematician	Described the state of health of the population, determinants of public health, as well as the application of the knowledge gained to the prevention and control of the disease	Mid-1800s
John Snow— physician	Established the cause and mode of communication of cholera in London	1854

Person	Contribution to Disease Causation	Time (Period)
British Medical Research Council	Streptomycin tuberculosis trial	1940s
Bradford Hill and Richard Doll	Established smoking as a causative agent in lung cancer	1950
Framingham Study	Foundation stone for cardiovascular risk factors (high blood pressure, elevated serum cholesterol level, physical activities, etc.)	1947–Present
Modern epidemiology	Health determinants at molecular and genetic levels; health determinants at biological and societal levels; penetration of the epidemiologic black box	21st century

Table 3-3   History of Modern Epidemiology *(continued)*

IV. **Models of Disease Causation [PHCC.3.3]**

   A. Causation refers to the process of an event (disease, disability, or injury) occurring as a result of either intrinsic or extrinsic factors acting individually or collectively.[4]

   B. Causal action of exposure comes before the subsequent development of disease as a consequence of exposure. Basis of longitudinal study where exposure data or information refers to an earlier time than that of disease, disability, or injury occurrence.[4]

   C. Intrinsic factor in disease causation simply refers to the host factor (organism). Example of this factor includes the immune system as well as the personality, social class membership, and race.

   D. The extrinsic factor refers to the environmental factors, which are identified as biological, social, and physical environments.[4,5]

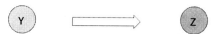

A. Necessary and sufficient conditions or factors in causal relationship

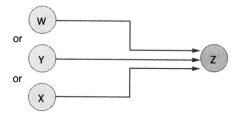

B. Sufficient but not necessary conditions or factors in causal relationship

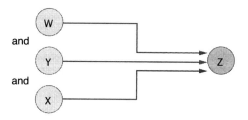

C. Necessary but not sufficient conditions or factors in causal relationship

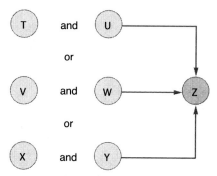

D. Neither sufficient nor necessary condition in causal relationship

Figure 3-1 Causal Relationships

Table 3-4 Models of Disease Causation	
Model	**Description**
Ecologic model	Disease occurs as a result of interrelationship between biological, social, and physical factors.
Epidemiologic triangle model*	Disease is caused by an imbalance between the host (intrinsic factor), agent, and environment.
Web of causation model	Diseases do not occur as a result of a single isolated factor but as a result of multiple factors interacting to predispose to disease (e.g., coronary artery disease, which is associated with diet, smoking, physical inactivity, estrogen replacement therapy, stress).
Wheel model (man/environment interaction)	This model stresses the genetic makeup as the most prominent determinant of a disease.
	Ignores agent in the causation of the disease and places gene at the core of disease causation as well as incorporates social, biological, and physical environment in the interpretation of disease process.
Causal pie (multi-causality)	Disease occurrence requires the joint action of component causes as "sufficient cause"; multitude of component causes.

* One of the most frequently used models, which claims that to understand the disease process, the environmental, the host, and the agent factors must be understood.

V.   **Measures of Disease Frequency**
   A. The measures of disease frequency include *ratios, proportion,* and *rates.*
   B. Rates as used in public health involve incident rates, mortality rates, attack rates, and fatality rates.
       1. The basic measures of disease frequency in epidemiology are incidence and prevalence.

C. *Ratio* is one number (*X*) divided by another (*Y*). For example, the sex of adults attending a blood pressure screening clinic could be compared in this way (e.g., male/female; male/male + female).

D. *Proportion:* It is a type of ratio, but the numerator is included in the denominator.

   1. The distinction between a ratio and proportion, therefore, implies that the proportion represents the relationship between *X* and *Y*.

E. *Rate* is a type of proportion and is a measure of occurrence of events in a population over time.

   1. Time is therefore an integral part of the denominator in rate.

   2. Rate = Number of cases or events occurring during a given time period / Population at risk during the same time period $\times 10^n$.

F. *Vignette:* During the first 12 months of Nostate surveillance for AIDS malignancy (AM), the Health Department received 2,166 case reports that specified sex; 1,000 cases were in females, 1,166 in males. How will you calculate the female-to-male ratio for AM? In addition, how will you calculate the proportion of males with AM?

   1. *Ratio computation:* (a) Identify the number of AM cases of female (*X*) and the number of AM cases of males (*Y*). (b) Compute the ratio by using the basic formula: *X* (cases in female) / *Y* (cases in males). (c) Substituting for *X* and *Y* → 1,000 / 1,166 = 0.86:1.

      a. Therefore, there was less than 1 female patient for each male patient who reported for AM to the Health Department.

   2. *Proportion computation:* (a) Identify the number of AM cases of females (*X*), and the number of AM cases of females and males (*Y*). (b) Compute the proportion by using the basic formula: *X* (cases in females) / *Y* (cases in females and males). (c) Substituting for *X* and *Y* → 1,000 / 2,166 = 0.46.

      a. Therefore, less than 5 out of every 10 AM cases were in females.

G. Ratios and proportions are used to characterize populations by age, sex, race, exposure, etc.

H. Rates, ratios, and proportions are used to describe morbidity, mortality, and natality health and human conditions.[4,6]

VI. Measures of Disease Occurrence [PHCC.3.5]

  A. Comparing disease frequency involves measuring disease occurrence.

  B. Measures of disease occurrence most frequently used in epidemiology are *risk, incidence rates,* and *prevalence.*[7]

  C. *Risk* refers to the probability that an individual or group of persons will develop a given disease.[6]

     1. If the total number of persons in a population (Notown) equals *T*, and *D* represents the number of people out of the *T* population who develop the disease (AM) during the period of time, the proportion *D / T* represents the average risk of developing AM in the population during that period.

  D. The *basic formula for risk* computation is: D / T = Number of subjects developing the disease or the event of interest during a time period / Number of subjects followed for that time period.

  E. The *average risk* of a disease in a population is interchangeable with the *incidence proportion* as well as the *cumulative incidence* (CI) of the disease.

     1. CI is the proportion of the population that becomes diseased or presents with the event of interest over a specified period of time.

     2. Average risk of getting a disease over a period of time, which is the probability of getting a disease.

     3. Adequate measure when there are small or no losses to follow up.

     4. The basic formula for CI is Number of new cases of disease or event of interest or related health factor / Number in the population of interest, over a specific time period.

  F. *Incidence rate* (IR) is the measure of disease frequency that utilizes cumulative incidence or average risk and ignores the concept of competing risk, thus underestimating the point estimate.[8,9]

  G. Rates can be used to estimate risk only when the period of follow-up is short and the rate of the disease over that interval is relatively constant.

     1. IR takes into account the competing risk by modeling the disease occurrence with the person-time (P-T) of observation.

  H. IR or *incidence density* (ID) is the occurrence of new cases of disease or events of interest that arise during P-T of observation.

1. The basic formula for IR is Number of subjects developing the disease or events of interest (new cases) / Total time experienced by the subjects followed (P-T) of observation.
2. *Vignette:* Consider that in Newcity, 35,000 women were at risk for postmenopausal breast cancer and contributed 250,000 person-years of follow-up. If there were 1,500 incident cases during the 10-year follow-up, what would be ID for breast cancer in this population?
3. *Computation:* (1) Identify the number of cases during the time period (*A*) and identify the total P-T of observation (follow-up) (*B*). (2) Apply the basic formula, *A* / *B*. (3) Substituting → 1,500 / 250,000 = 600.0 per 100,000 per year.
4. *Cumulative incidence* is related to *incidence rate* by the formula CI = IR × *T*, where *T* is the specified period of time.
5. Risk is related to IR and is mathematically given by Risk = IR × *T*.

I. *Prevalence proportion* (P) measures the frequency of the existing disease (disease status).
  1. Two types of prevalence measures are common in epidemiology:
     a. *Point prevalence* (proportion of the population that is diseased (new cases, current cases, old cases) at a single point in time).
     b. *Period prevalence* (proportion of the population that is diseased during a specified duration of time), for example, during the year 2006.
J. The denominator for the point prevalence is the estimated population at the point in time, whereas the denominator of the period prevalence is the estimated population at mid-interval.
K. *Prevalence* is influenced by *time.*
  1. The longer the duration of the disease, the greater the prevalence.
  2. Prevalence is influenced by both IR and disease duration.
  3. The relationship between prevalence and IR is given by P = IR × *D*, where *D* is the duration of the disease or the event of interest (applicable to low disease prevalence, i.e., less than 10%).

L. When the prevalence of the disease is not low, the relationship between the prevalence and IR is given by $ID / 1 + ID$, where $I =$ incidence and $D =$ the duration of the disease.

1. The basic formula for *point prevalence* is Number of existing cases of disease or event of interest / Number in total population, at the point in time.

2. *Period prevalence* is given by the formula Number of existing cases of disease or event of interest / Number in total population (estimated population at mid-interval).

VII. Uses of Incidence and Prevalence Data

Table 3-5   Uses of Incidence and Prevalence Data in Public Health

Prevalence

Important and useful in the planning and monitoring of public health services (facilities, personnel, manpower)

Expresses the burden of health-related events in a specified population

Useful in determining the extent of the health-related events

Substitution for the calculation of the impact of the health-related events in the absence of incidence data

 ▪ Not a good estimator of incidence

Point prevalence is useful in tracking changes of health-related events in a population over time

Incidence

Important in estimating disease etiology

Provides direct measure of disease/disability/injury rate or risk

Allows for hypothesis testing on the magnitude of the effect of the risk factor(s) on the outcome of the health-related event (disease/disability/injury)

VIII. Limitations of Prevalence Data in Public Health [PHCC.3.5]

A. Tends to produce biased picture of the health-related events such as disease, favoring the inclusion of chronic over acute diseases.

B. Cause and effect are measured simultaneously.

C. Cannot be used for causal inference.

D. Determined from one survey, whereas incidence requires at least two sets of observations (records/data) of the same subject.

IX. **Types of Rates (Crude, Specific, Adjusted) [PHCC.3.5]**

   A. *Crude rates* are based on the actual number of events in a population over a given time period.

      1. Examples of crude rates are birth rate, infant mortality rate, fetal death rate, maternal mortality rate, etc.

   B. Crude birth rate is computed by the basic formula Number of live births within a given period / Population size at the middle of that period × 1,000 population.

      1. *Vignette:* Consider a population of Newcountry to be 280,000,000 during 1996, and the number of babies born was 4,500,000 during the same period.

      2. The crude birth rate will be Number of live births (*A*) / Population size (*B*) × 1,000. Substituting for *A* and *B* → 4,500,000 / 280,000,000 × 1,000 = 16.07 per 1,000.

Table 3-6   Crude Rates: Example and Basic Formula for Rate Estimation

Crude Rate	Formula	Interpretation
Birth rate	Number of live births within a given period / Population size at the middle of that period × 1,000 population	Projects population changes Affected by number of women of childbearing age
Infant mortality	Number of infant deaths among infants aged 0 to 365 days during the year / Number of live births during the year × 1,000 live births	Used for international comparison Low rates reflect balanced health needs
Post-neonatal mortality rate	Number of infant deaths from 28 to 365 days after birth / Number of live births minus neonatal deaths × 1,000 live births	Low rates reflect environmental events, infectious disease control, and adequate nutrition

---

   C. The rate is often incorrectly used to refer to proportions or ratios, as in these illustrations.

   D. *Vignette:* Consider a population of 200,000 people of whom 40 are diagnosed with pancreatic neoplasm (PN) in 2005, and during the same time period (2005), 36 died from PN. How will you calculate the mortality rate in 2005 in this population, and the case fatality rate in this population?

1. *Computation:* (a) Mortality rate as a result of PN: 36 / 200,000 = 0.00018 (0.018%) or 18.0 per 100,000. (b) Case fatality as a result of PN: 36 / 40 = 0.9 (90%).

E. *Specific rates* refer to a particular subgroup of the population defined such as age, sex, social class, and race. Example of specific rate is age-specific rate.

F. Age-specific rate refers to the number of cases per age group of population during a specified time period.

1. *Vignette:* Consider that in Nocounty during 2006, there were 1,100 deaths due to bronchial carcinoma (BC) among the 55–74 age group, and there were 35,000,000 persons in that age group. What will be the age-specific BC death rate in this age group?

2. *Computation:* Using the formula Number of deaths (BC) among those aged 55–74 years (A) / Number of persons aged 55–74 years during 2006 (B) × 100,000. Substituting → A / B × 100,000; 1,100 / 35,000,000 × 100,000 = 3.14 per 100,000.

G. *Adjusted rates* refers to summary measures of the rate of morbidity and mortality in a population in which statistical procedures have been applied to remove the effect of differences in the composition of the various populations such as age for the purpose of comparison.

H. Two methods of rate adjustment are most commonly used in public health:

1. *Direct method* is used if age-specific death rates in a population to be standardized are known and a suitable standard population is available.

2. *Indirect method,* or standardized mortality ratio (SMR), is used when the age-specific death rates are unknown or unstable.

I. *Direct method:* (1) Multiply the age-specific rate by the number of persons. (2) Sum the expected number of deaths in each age group to determine the total number of expected deaths. (3) The age-adjusted rate is Total expected number of deaths / Number of deaths in the standardized or combined population, × 100,000.

1. The result, the adjusted death rate, ensures that the observed differences in the death rates between the two populations compared are not due to age, gender, or sex.

2. *Vignette:* Using Table 3–7, consider the age group in years, the age-specific death rates per 100,000 in Populations X and Y, and the number in the United States in 1998 (census population estimates). Determine which population has excess mortality.

Table 3-7   Age-Specific Mortality Rates for Populations X and Y

Age Group	(A) Population X (Age-specific rates per 100,000)	(B) Population Y (Age-specific rates per 100,000)	(C) U.S. Population (1998 Census estimate)	(D) (Expected deaths for population X)	(E) (Expected deaths for population Y)
< 5 years	149.19	181.40	18,989,257		
5–19	43.44	36.78	58,712,947		
20–24	165.97	178.23	100,919,429		
45–64	521.18	725.04	57,241,131		
> 65 years	4,011.94	4,517.68	34,385,239		
Total	417.91	1,060.94	270,248,003		

Source: Data from National Center for Health Statistics, Division of Data Services.

3. *Computation:* (a) Multiply A by C to obtain D, expected deaths for population X. (b) Multiply B and C to obtain E, expected deaths for population Y. (c) Obtain the age adjusted rate for population X by summing the total in column D and dividing by the total in column C, then multiplying by 100,000. (d) Repeat these steps for population Y. (e) Subtract the rate in X (702.56 per 100,000) from Y (815.15 per 100.000). The excess age-adjusted mortality rate is 112.6 per 100,000.

J. *Indirect age-adjusted rate* (SMR) is calculated by Observed number of deaths (A) / Expected number of deaths (B) × 100.

1. *Vignette:* Consider the number of observed deaths in Notown from angina pectoris to be 1,200 during 2005. If the expected number of death is 2,000, what is the SMR?

2. *Computation*: SMR = $A / B \times 100$. Substituting → 1,200 / 2,000 = 0.6 (60%).

X. **Measures of Disease Comparison [PHCC.3.5]**

  A. *Absolute*

    1. Subtracted from one another.

    2. Provide information about public health impact of an exposure.

  B. *Relative*

    1. Divided from one another.

    2. Provide information about the strength of the relationship between exposure (independent variable) and outcome (disease, disabilities, or injuries).

  C. Absolute measures of comparison are risk difference, rate difference, IR difference, CI difference, and prevalence difference.

  D. Relative measures of comparison are risk ratio, rate ratio, relative rate or relative risk, IR ratio, CI ratio, and prevalence ratio.

  E. *Rate versus risk*

    1. Risk is the accumulated effect of rate occurring during some specified time period.

    2. Risk has no time dimension, and the reference population in risk is the population unaffected at the beginning of the period of observation.

BOX 3-1   CAUSE-SPECIFIC RATES

- Cause-specific death rate is the most commonly used cause-specific rate.
- Cause-specific death rate is given by: Number of death due to a particular cause (place and time defined) / Mid-period population (same place and time period) $\times$ 1,000.
- The underling causes of death is assumed to be provided by the death certificates.
- Advantage-provided information on trends in causes of death over time, as well as useful information on disease relationship with respect to the burden of disease in the population.
- Limitations—not accurate for causal factors.

F. *Attack rate* (AR), although not specifically a rate but a proportion, is the CI of a disease during an outbreak or transient epidemic.[4,7]
   1. AR = Diseased (exposed and developed an illness) / Diseased and Nondiseased (all exposed to the suspected agent of contamination) × (multiplier [100]) during a time period.

G. *Secondary attack rate* (SAR) is the proportion of individuals exposed to the primary case (primary cases), who themselves develop the disease (secondary case).[4]
   1. SAR = Number of new cases in group minus − Initial case(s) / Number of susceptible persons in a group − Initial case(s).

H. *Vignette:* Consider data on primary and secondary attack from salmonella pathogen. Is this a rate or ratio?
   1. *Solution:* Because time is not involved in the denominator, this measure of disease is strictly not a rate but a risk (proportion).

Table 3-8	Measures of Comparison	
Measure	**Formula**	**Explanation**
Rate or risk ratio	RE/RU, where RE = risk or rate in the exposed and RU = risk or rate in the unexposed	Measures the strength of association between exposure and the disease (outcome)
Attributable proportion among total population	$(RT - RU)/RT \times 100$, where RT = incidence rate (IR), cumulative incidence (CI), or prevalence proportion (PP) in the total population and RU is the IR, CI, or PP in the unexposed population	Measures the excess proportion of disease in the total population, assuming the exposure is causal and implying the proportion of a disease in a total population that will be eliminated if the exposure were eliminated
Attributable proportion among the exposed	$(RE - RU)/RE \times 100$	Measures the proportion of disease among the exposed, assuming the exposure is causal and implying the

Table 3-8	Measures of Comparison *(continued)*	
Measure	**Formula**	**Explanation**
		proportion of disease among the exposed that will be eliminated if the exposure is eliminated
Population rate difference	$RT - RU$ or $RD \times PE$, where $RD =$ IR difference, CI difference, or PP difference; and $PE =$ proportion of population that is exposed, and $RD = RE - RU$	Measures excess rate or risk of a disease or outcome in the total population
Rate or risk difference	$RE - RU$	Measures rate or risk of disease or outcome among the exposed population
Attack rate	ND / TP, where $ND =$ number of people at risk in whom a certain outcome develops, and $TP =$ total number of people at risk	Compares the risk of outcome in groups with different exposure

XI. Sources of Epidemiologic Data [PHCC.3.4]

Table 3-9	Sources of Epidemiologic Data
Sources	**Description**
Vital statistics	Provides information for births, deaths, marriages, and divorces
U.S. Census	Provides information on complete counts of U.S. population every 10 years
	Types of information include race, sex, age, and marital status (all samples) and income, education level, housing, and occupation (representative samples)

Table 3-9 Sources of Epidemiologic Data (continued)	
Sources	**Description**
National Health Interview Survey	Provides data on major health problems, such as acute and chronic disease conditions, impairment and injuries, and utilization of the health services, such as dental care
	Useful in examining annual changes in disease and disabilities conditions
National Health and Nutrition Examination Survey (NHANES)	Provides information on the health and diet of the U.S. population based on home interview and nutritional examination
Behavioral Risk Factor Surveillance System	Survey of random sample of U.S. population by phone interviews on behaviors affecting health and well-being (exercise, smoking, obesity, alcohol, automobile seat belts, and drinking and driving)
National Notifiable Disease Surveillance System	Provides information on most communicable diseases, including HIV/AIDS, botulism, gonorrhea, human and animal rabies, etc.
Surveillance, Epidemiology, and End Results Program (SEER)	National Cancer Institute database that provides information on trends in cancer incidence, mortality, and survival
	Information includes patient demographics, primary cancer sites, pathology, first mode of therapy, and severity of the disease
World Health Statistics Annual	Provides information on international morbidity and mortality
Cancer Incidence of Five Continents	WHO's international agency for research and cancer that provides information on cancer incidence and mortality globally (estimated 170 cancer registries in 50 countries)
National occupational hazards survey and national occupational exposure survey	Provides data on workers exposed to chemical, physical, and biologic agents
Surveillance of AIDS and HIV infection	Provides information on HIV/AIDS incidence and prevalence, as well as cumulative incidence

XII. **Epidemiologic Study Designs (Experimental and Observational) [PHCC.3.5, 3.6]**

A. Designs in epidemiologic investigations may be observational (the investigator does not manipulate the assignment of subjects) or experimental (subjects are randomized to the various arms of treatment or placebo).

B. Epidemiologic designs commonly used are *ecologic, case-control/comparison, cross-sectional* (prevalence), *cohort* (longitudinal), *retrospective cohort* (historical/nonconcurrent prospective study), *prospective cohort* (concurrent/concurrent prospective), and *experimental* (randomized trial).[2,9]

C. The main goal of analytic design is to determine whether there is an association between the factors or characteristics and the development of a disease, disabilities, or injuries.

D. If association exists, design also allows one to derive appropriate inferences regarding a potential causal relationship.

E. Analysis could be at the individual level as in cross-sectional study, case-control study, cohort study, and clinical trials.

F. Analysis could also be at the group level, for example, ecologic design. (Be conscious of ecologic fallacy, which claims that an association occurs at individual level when the analysis was performed at a group level.)

G. *Ecologic design*

1. An observational epidemiologic study design.

2. Examines the relationship between exposure and the outcome of interest (disease, disability, and injury) with population level rather than the individual level as a unit of data gathering and analysis.

3. Correlation coefficient is the point estimate for the measure of association.

4. Limitations include the inability to establish temporal sequence and the tendency to make cross-level inferences from group to individual (ecologic fallacy).

H. *Cross-sectional design*

Table 3-10   Cross-Sectional (Prevalence) Design: Description, Measure of Association, Strengths, and Limitations

Description
- Snapshots of a population at a single point in time.
- Defines a population and determines the presence or absence of exposure and the presence or absence of disease for each subject.

Measure of association
- Measure of the exposure prevalence in relation to disease, disability, or injury prevalence.
- Using a 2 × 2 table, the prevalence of the disease in the exposed: $a/a + b$; presence of the disease in subjects without exposure: $c/c + d$; prevalence of exposure in persons with the disease: $a/a + c$, and prevalence of exposure in subjects without disease: $b/b + d$.
- Prevalence risk/odds ratio: $a/(a + b)/c/(c + d)$; where a = exposed and diseased, b = exposed and non-diseased, c = unexposed but diseased, and d = unexposed and nondiseased.

Strengths and advantages
- Generalizability.
- Inexpensive.

Limitations
- Inability to assess temporal sequence between exposure and disease or health-related events if exposure changes over time (not possible to tell whether the exposure preceded the development of disease).
- Preponderance of prevalent cases of long duration.
- Healthy worker survival effects (association may be due to survival after the health-related event rather than with the risk of development of health-related event).

Vignettes
- Consider a study that is interested in the possible association between low serum lycopene level (exposure) and prostate cancer (disease). If the population is surveyed and the serum lycopene is determined for all subjects, perform prostate specific antigen for prostate cancer, and both exposure and disease are determined at the same time.
   a) Could this constitute a cross-sectional design?
   b) Calculate the prevalence risk ratio if 20 of the 60 men with low serum lycopene level had prostate cancer while 10 of the 80 men with high serum lycopene level had prostate cancer.
- *Computing*: Prevalence risk ratio: $a/(a + b)/c/(c + d)$. Substituting →
   (20 / 80) / (10 / 90) = 0.25 / 0.11 = 2.27.

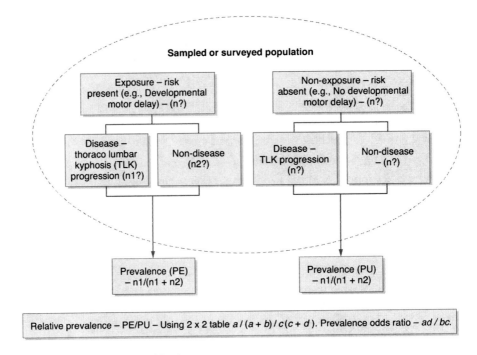

Figure 3-2   Cross-Sectional Design

I. *Case-control or comparison design*

Description

- Method of sampling a population in which epidemiologists (investigators) identify and enroll cases of disease or health-related event and a sample of the source population that produced the cases.

- Hallmark of case-control study is that it begins with the disease (cases) and compares them with people without disease (control).[2,7,9]

- Compares a group of individuals who have experienced the outcome (health-related event) under study (cases) with a group who have not (control or comparison).

- Cases are identified (formulation of a disease or case definition) as to whether they belong to exposed or unexposed group (cohort), whereas the control is sampled from the source population.

Table 3-11   Case-Control Design: Description, Measure of Association, Strengths, and Limitations *(continued)*

- The control group is used to estimate the distribution of the exposure in the source population; control must be sampled independently of the exposure status.
- Variant designs:
  - *Case-crossover*, a design where cases serve as their own controls; is appropriate in settings in which the risk of the outcome is increased for only a brief time following exposure (typical exposure is something that varies from time to time within an individual).[6,9] Uses the previous experience of the cases as a substitute for control series to estimate the person-time distribution in the source population.
  - *Nested case-control*, a hybrid design where new case controls are derived from a cohort study (nested) of the original design.[2,6]
  - *Case-cohort*, study in which every person in the source population has the same chance of being included as a control, regardless of the time contributed by that person to the person-time experience of the cohort.[2,6]

Measure of association

- Using a 2 × 2 table, the sample of all available cases $= (a + c)$, and independently, a sample of unaffected subjects (comparison/control) $= (b + d)$.
- The primary measure of association is odds ratio or relative odds, which is simply the cross-products ratio.
- Odds ratio (OR) is calculated by multiplying the number opposite it on the diagonal of the 2 × 2 table, and this result is then divided by the two other numbers multiplied together (cross-products ratio).
- $OR = (a/b)/(c/d) \rightarrow ad/bc$ (cross products).[2,10]
- *Odds concept*: The odds that the case was exposed: a/c; whereas the odds that a control was exposed: b/d. The odds ratio is simply the ratio that the cases were exposed to the odds that the controls were exposed: $(a/c) \div (b/d)$. Therefore OR = (product of diseased people exposed and non-diseased people unexposed) ad / (product of non-diseased people exposed and diseased people unexposed) $bc \rightarrow OR = ad/bc$.

Strengths and advantages

- Efficient for rare diseases (desirable design).
- Efficient for diseases with long induction and latent periods.

Table 3-11 Case-Control Design: Description, Measure of Association, Strengths, and Limitations *(continued)*

- Adequate for evaluating multiple exposures in relation to a disease (desirable when little is known about exposure variables in a given disease).
- Rapid and inexpensive relative to prospective cohort design.

Limitations

- Recall and selection bias. Recall bias due to the retrospective nature of the design.[2,9]
- Difficult to assess temporal sequence between exposure and disease or health-related events if exposure changes over time.[6]
- Information bias and poor information on exposure (retrospective nature of the design).
- Inefficient for rare exposure.

Vignette

- Consider a study that is interested in the possible association between smoking (exposure) and coronary heart disease [CHD] (disease). If the investigators begin with 400 people with CHD (cases) and compare them with 800 controls (people without CHD), is this a case-control investigation? Suppose 224 of the 400 cases were smokers and 176 were nonsmokers. Of the 800 controls, 352 were smokers and 448 were nonsmokers.

  a. What is the measure of association in this investigation, and how could this be calculated?

- *Computing:* The exposure odds ratio: *ad/bc*. Substituting → 224 × 448 ÷ 176 × 352 = 1.62. This result indicates that individuals with smoking history had a 62% increased risk of experiencing CHD compared to those with no history of smoking.

1. Note: (a) Because the two groups are sampled separately, rates of disease, disabilities, or injuries in the exposed or unexposed groups cannot be calculated, nor can relative risk be measured directly. However, the odds ratio can be computed, which is the primary measure of association in case-control design. (b) Because of the sampling used, the total number exposed is not *a* + *b*, and the risk in exposed subjects is not *a* / (*a* + *b*).

2. Nested case-control is advantageous to the classic case-control in that (a) it minimizes and eliminates recall bias; (b) it

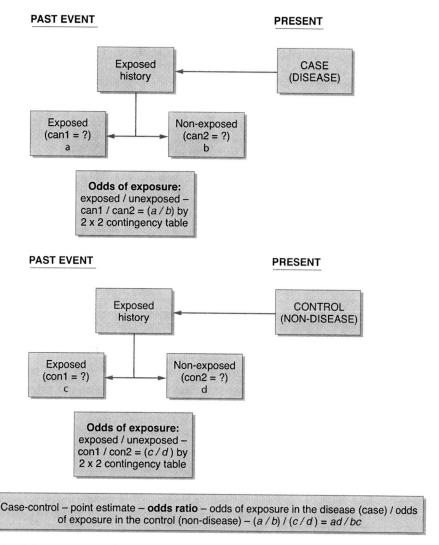

Figure 3-3 Case-Control Design

ensures or reduces temporal sequence, thus making it easy to determine whether the exposure preceded the disease; and (c) it is relatively inexpensive and rapid, compared to prospective cohort design.[9]

3. Nested case control is limited in that the nondiseased may not be fully representative of the original cohort due to loss to follow-up or death.

4. Odds ratio is a good estimate of relative risk, except when the outcome is very frequent (high prevalence).

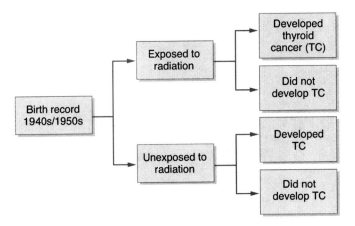

Figure 3-4   Retrospective Cohort Design

5. *Odds and probability (case-control versus cohort design):* Odds differs from probability (P) but is related by: Odds = P ÷ (1 − P). For example, if the probability of disease being exposed is 80% (0.8), the odds of disease being exposed is 4.0, which is 80 / 20 (P / 1 − P).

   a. In a cohort design, the probability that the exposed will develop a disease is $a / a + b$ and the odds that a disease will develop in the exposed is a / b (P / 1 − P). The probability that the disease will develop in the unexposed is $c / c + d$; similarly, the odds of disease developing in the unexposed is c / d (P / 1 − P).

BOX 3-2   STUDY DESIGNS: CROSS-SECTIONAL VERSUS CASE-CONTROL

- *Cross-sectional* studies, also termed surveys, and prevalence studies are designed to assess both the exposure and outcome simultaneously.
- However, since exposure and disease status are measured at the same point in time (snapshot), it is difficult, if not impossible, to distinguish whether the exposure preceded or followed the disease, and thus cause and effect relationships are not certain, lacking temporal sequence.
- A *case-control design* classifies subjects on the basis of outcome (disease and non-disease or comparison group) and then looks backward to identify the exposure.
- This design could be prospective as well.
- In this design, the history or previous events for both cases and comparison groups are assessed in an attempt to identify the exposure or risk factors for the disease.

      b. The odds ratio *(incidence rate ratio)* in cohort design *is a / b ÷ c / d = ad / bc*, which is the odds that an exposed person develops a disease divided by the odds that a nonexposed person develops a disease.

J. *Cohort design*

Table 3-12   Cohort Design: Description, Measure of Association, Strengths, and Limitations

Description

- Design that represents a group of individuals who are followed over a period of time for the occurrence of a specific disease(s), disability, or injury.
- Typically comprises two cohorts, namely, exposed and unexposed.
- The purpose of follow-up is to measure the occurrence of the health-related event(s), with the aim of comparing the specific disease(s), disability, or injury rates for two or more cohorts.
- Two cohorts are commonly followed in epidemiology: (1) *closed* (fixed membership—allows no addition of individual once follow-up begins), example, randomized clinical trial, and (2) *open* (dynamic cohort that can take new members as time passes), example, state cancer registry that comprises the state residents and is dynamic because new residents may be added to the registry.
- The study group is the exposed, while the comparison is the unexposed.

Measure of association

- Risk or incidence can be estimated from a closed cohort. Please note that the computation of risk is complicated by competing risk—the removal of some subjects from the population at risk before they have experienced the entire follow-up period.
- Risk can be estimated directly if there is (1) a short follow-up period (< 30 days) or (2) a small competing risk (very few or no deaths).
- Under this assumption (short follow-up period and no competing risk), risk is estimated by dividing the number of new health-related events by the total number of people being followed (population at risk) in the closed cohort.
- Incidence rate (IR) calculation is the appropriate measure and a more reliable estimate if the cohort is dynamic. Therefore, one must take into account the amount of time each person contributes as a member of the population at risk in addressing competing risk in the dynamic as well as close cohort that is designated with a long follow-up period and competing risks.

Table 3-12   Cohort Design: Description, Measure of Association, Strengths, and Limitations *(continued)*

- IR is computed by dividing the number of new cases (incident cases) by the amount of person-time experienced by the population at risk.
- *Computation*: Relative risk (RR) $= a/a + b$ (incidence in the exposed) $\div$ $c/c + d$ (incidence in the unexposed). Where the denominator is the person-time, the RR represents the incidence rate (IR) or incidence density (ID).
- *RR interpretation*: (1) RR $= 1.0$ (no association—null), (2) RR > 1.0 (positive association—predisposing/possibly causal), or (3) RR < 1.0 (negative association—protective).

Strengths and advantages

- Efficient for rare exposure.
- Establishes a clear temporal relationship between exposure and the outcome of interest (prospective design).
- Particularly efficient for diseases with long induction and latent periods (retrospective design).
- Produces a direct measure of risk or incidence of disease.
- Produces reliable information on exposures, especially prospective designs.
- Appropriate in assessing multiple effects of an exposure.
- Feasible relative to experimental design when ethical consideration precludes such conduct (less vulnerable to ethical restrictions of randomized clinical trials).

Limitations

- Relatively expensive compared to case-control or cross-sectional design.
- Takes long time to conduct (loss to follow-up, change of exposure over time $\rightarrow$ exposure misclassification $\rightarrow$ attenuation of the point estimate [RR]).
- Inefficient for diseases with long induction and latent periods (prospective design).
- Inefficient for rare outcomes (prospective design).
- Vulnerable to information and other types of bias (selection, misclassification)—retrospective design.
- Minimal information on exposure and some key variables, restricting controlling for confounders due to unmeasured confounding $\rightarrow$ biased point estimate (retrospective design).

Table 3-12   Cohort Design: Description, Measure of Association, Strengths, and Limitations *(continued)*

Vignette

- Consider a cohort study to compare the mortality rate of myocardial infarction (MI) in men with sedentary work (exposed group) to men with physically active work (unexposed). If in the exposed, there were 18,000 person (man)-years of observation and 63 deaths; whereas the unexposed had 12,000 man-years of observation and 22 deaths.

    a. What will the mortality rate be in each cohort?

    b. What is the relative risk/incidence density of dying, comparing these two groups?

    c. What is the attributable risk of sedentary work?

    d. What is the attributable benefit of physical activity?

    e. If we assume that MI is associated with the mortality in this cohort (causality), what proportion of disease in the higher risk group is potentially preventable?

Computation

- (a) *Mortality rate* in each cohort (1) Exposed group → Number of deaths among those in the sedentary group (exposed) / Person-time experience → 63 / 18,000 = 0.0035 (multiplier − 100,000) → 0.0035 × 100,000 = 350 deaths per 100,000 man-years; (2) using the same basic formula in (1) and substituting: 22 / 12,000 → 0.0018 (multiplier − 100,000) → 0.0018 × 100,000 = 183 deaths per 100,000 man-years.

- (b) *Relative risk*: Risk in the exposed / Risk in the unexposed → 350 / 183 per 100,000 man-years = 1.91.

- (c) *Attributable risk* (risk difference) of sedentary work: Risk in the exposed − Risk in the unexposed → 350 − 183 deaths per 100,000 →167 deaths per 100,000 man-years.

- (d) *Attributable benefit* of physical activity simply implies the risk difference → 167 deaths per 100,000.

- (e) *Attributable proportion* in the exposed = Attributable risk (*A*) / Total risk in the exposed (*B*). Also, (RR -1) / (RR).

- *Substituting*: A / B = 167 / 350 per 100,000 man-years → 47.7%. Thus, the preventable proportion as a result of eliminating sedentary lifestyle in the exposed group will be 47.7% of deaths due to MI in this group.

1. *Desirability of cohort designs*
   a. Use cohort design (prospective) when: (1) multiple effects of exposure are assessed or (2) exposure is rare.
   b. Use cohort design (retrospective) when (1) outcome of interest has long induction period, (2) outcome of interest has a long latent period, or (3) outcome is rare.
2. *Types of cohort designs:*
   a. *Prospective:* Study subjects are selected on the basis of exposure and followed over time.

BOX 3-3   TRADITIONAL COHORT DESIGNS—PROSPECTIVE VERSUS RETROSPECTIVE

- Cohort studies are traditionally classified as (a) prospective and (b) retrospective, depending on the temporal relationship between the initiation of the study and the outcome (occurrence of disease or event of interest).
- A design is considered a retrospective cohort, which also is termed historical cohort or nonconcurrent prospective study, if the exposures and the outcomes of interest (disease, for example) have already occurred prior to the initiation of the study.
- In prospective design, the exposure, which defines the cohort, has occurred in the exposed group prior to the initiation of the study but the outcome (disease) has not occurred.
- In this context, both groups are followed to assess the incidence rate of the disease, comparing the exposed to the unexposed.
- However, the main distinction between these two designs is the calendar time.
- For example, if exposure to radiation is ascertained from birth data (medical record) and the outcome (thyroid cancer) at the beginning of the study (no follow-up), then the design is retrospective cohort.

---

   b. *Retrospective:* Both the exposure and outcome of interest have already occurred prior to the commencement of study.
   c. *Ambirectional:* Cohort study with both prospective and retrospective components.

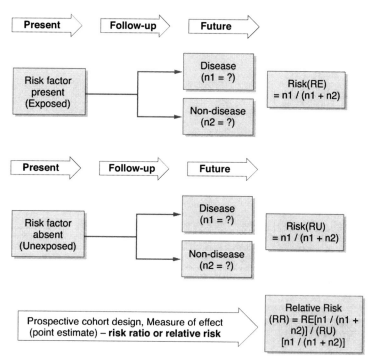

Figure 3-5   Prospective Cohort Design

BOX 3-4   BASIC DISTINCTIONS OF EPIDEMIOLOGIC STUDY DESIGNS

- A design that begins with exposure(s) of interest and disease-free subjects, and aimed to assess the outcome in future by following the subjects represents a *prospective cohort study*.
- The time relation in prospective cohort study is present and future (continuing).
- A *case-crossover design* uses the previous experience of the cases as a substitute for a control series, to estimate the person-time distribution in the source population.
- *Ambidirectional cohort* is a design that is both retrospective and prospective in its observation of the outcome.
- *Retrospective cohort* (historical cohort studies) is a design in which the cohorts are identified from recorded information and the time during which they are at risk for disease occurred before the beginning of the study.
- Simply, retrospective study is conducted by defining the cohort and collecting information which applies to past time.
- *Case-Control* is a design in which the groups of individuals are defined in terms of whether they have or have not already experienced the outcome under consideration, and the exposure is then measured.

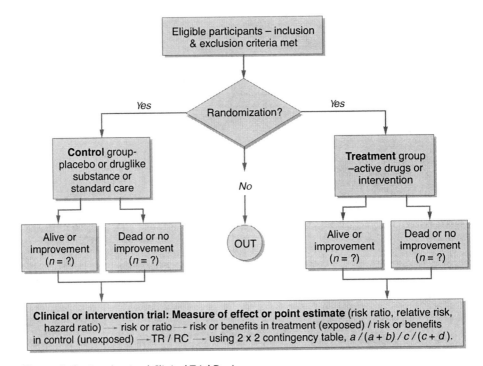

Figure 3-6 Randomized Clinical Trial Design

K. *Experimental design*

BOX 3-5 BASICS OF EXPERIMENTAL DESIGNS

- Experimental design, if feasible, is considered the gold standard compared with observational studies.
- The active manipulation or assignment of the treatment by the investigator is the hallmark that differentiates experimental designs from observational studies.
- Whereas not all experimental designs utilize blindness to minimize bias, blindness is not a feature of observational designs.
- Neither in observational design nor experimental ones are investigators required to manipulate the outcome.
- Experimental designs, like observational ones, are conducted in human as well as animal populations.

Table 3-13   Experimental Designs: Description, Measure of Association, Strengths, and Limitations

Description

- Nonobservational and involves random assignment of subjects to treatment and control groups.
- Best design of studying new interventions on individual or community basis.
- Prospective in time relationship.
- Gold standard of epidemiologic investigation when feasible; allows randomized double-blinded placebo-control assessment.

Measure of association

- Same as prospective cohort study (relative risk, odds ratio, hazard ratio).
- Unlike prospective cohort, the analysis to yield the point estimate could be:

  (a) *Intent-to-treat analysis* (data on the effectiveness of treatment under everyday practice condition; all randomized subjects whether or not there is an assurance on treatment compliance).[9]

  (b) *Efficacy analysis* (data on treatment effects under ideal condition).

Strengths and advantages

- Randomization—most appropriate way to control confounding.
- Double blinded—most appropriate way to control bias.
- Provides direct measure of association for benefits or risk (relative risk, risk ratio, hazard ratio).

Limitations

- Loss to follow-up (prospective), especially in long-term trials involving many years of follow-up.
- Generalizability—efficacy treatment may not necessarily translate to effectiveness of the treatment in real-world situations (community settings).
- Ethical consideration—patients cannot be assigned to exposure with known adverse effects, such as tobacco ingestion.[6,9]

Vignette 1

- Consider a clinical trial of 2,000 subjects (close cohort) with angina pectoris of whom half (1,000, intervention/treatment) received Nitroglycerin-G2 (new drug) and the other half (1,000, control) received the standard therapy (Nitroglycerin). After 5 years of follow-up, 200 deaths were reported in the intervention group and 350 from the control. If we assume nondifferential loss to follow-up or no loss in the two arms, what is the relative mortality associated with the new drug? What is your interpretation of the result?

Table 3-13   Experimental Designs: Description, Measure of Association, Strengths, and Limitations *(continued)*

- *Computation:* (1) Mortality rate in the intervention = Number of deaths / Population at risk. Substituting → 200 / 1,000 = 0.2 (20%). (2) Mortality rate in the control = Number of deaths (control group) / Population at risk (control group). Substituting → 350 / 1,000 = 0.35 (35%). (3) Relative mortality associated with the new drug = Rate in the intervention group / Rate in the control group. Substituting → 0.2 / 0.35 = 0.57.

- *Interpretation:* Relative risk less than 1.0 is indicative of the protective effect of the new drug with respect to mortality in the intervention population compared to the control.

Vignette 2

- Consider a clinical trial of Bacillus Calmette-Guerin vaccination in which 556 children were vaccinated and 8 died and 528 were not (control) and 8 died. Assuming this was a randomized clinical trial, what is the relative risk of dying? Is the vaccine protective against dying compared with the placebo (control)?

- *Computation:* (1) Mortality rate in the vaccinated = Number of deaths in the vaccinated group / Population at risk (vaccinated children). Substituting → 8 / 556 = 0.014 (1.44%). (2) Mortality rate in the control group = Number of deaths in the control group / Population at risk (control). Substituting → 8 / 528 = 0.015 (1.51%). Relative risk = Rate in the vaccinated children / Rate in the control. Substituting → 1.44 / 1.51 = 0.95.

- *Interpretation:* The relative risk less than 1.0 (null − no association) is indicative of the benefit of the vaccine in decreasing mortality in the vaccinated group compared with the control.

1. *Types of experimental trial:* (a) cross-over (each group receives all treatment but not simultaneously), (b) parallel (each group receives one treatment but treatments are administered concurrently), (c) simple (each group receives only one treatment), (d) factorial (each group receives two or more treatments), (e) community, (f) individual, (g) preventive, and (h) therapeutic.[9]

> **BOX 3-6   ANALYSIS STRATEGIES IN INTERVENTION TRIAL**
> - Analysis strategies in intervention trial—intent to treat versus efficacy analysis.
> - Two types of analytic approaches are often used in clinical trials (randomized), namely efficacy and intent-to-treat.
> - The latter is a method of analysis used in which all patients randomly assigned to one of the treatments arms are analyzed together, regardless of whether or not they completed or received that treatment.
> - On the other hand, efficacy analysis is performed only on those who comply with the assigned treatment.

2. *Double blinded:* Neither the experimental nor the study subjects have knowledge of the intervention assignment.
3. *Placebo control:* The control group is given an inactive treatment (water pill/nondrug), which resembles the intervention drug.

L. *Meta-analytic design (quantitative systematic review)*
1. Method of combining the results from a number of studies of similar design to produce an overall estimate of effect, which incorporates the information provided by all the studies.
   a. Popular method of critically assessing the value of evidence used to support health interventions—evidence-based medicine, quantitative evidence synthesis.
   b. Useful in answering research questions whenever an investigation of a particular research subject presents with conflicting or contradictory results. For example, some research groups may report a statistically significant difference in the use of anti-androgen in prolonging survival of men treated for loco-regional prostate cancer (CaP) while other groups report no statistically significant difference.
   c. A method of summarizing, integrating, and interpreting research studies that produces quantitative findings.
   d. A technique of encoding and analyzing the statistics that summarize research findings.
2. If full data sets of studies of interest are available, a pool analysis is the preferred method.
3. Because meta-analysis focuses on the aggregation and comparison of findings of different research studies, meaningful

comparability is required. For example, studies assessing the association between selenium intake and CaP can be compared with meta-analytic design using prospective cohort or case-control studies but not mixed, given the differences in the point estimates generated by these two designs. Likewise, observational and experimental cannot be mixed in meta-analytic designs but can be compared separately.[11]

4. Meta-analysis represents each study's findings in the form of effect sizes or point estimates. An effect size encodes the quantitative information from each relevant study's findings. Studies that produce bivariate correlations cannot be combined with those that compared groups of subjects on the mean values of the dependent variables.

5. *Methodology:* This involves (a) defining the research question, (b) defining the criteria for studies to be included, (c) identifying and retrieving the studies that meet the inclusion criteria, (d) abstracting information, (e) analyzing statistics (fixed effect or random-effect analysis), and (f) reporting results.

6. *Statistical/analytic methods:* Fixed and random effect models.

7. *Heterogeneity test:* Tests whether the overall summary estimate is an adequate representation of the dataset; compares each of the individual study results with the summary estimate; examines the differences between the studies. Based on weighted average of the difference of the results of each study and the summary estimate of the effect. If there is significant heterogeneity, the analysis may be repeated after excluding the studies that are particularly divergent. The heterogeneity statistics produce an χ^2 value for each individual study, based on the comparison of that study's result to the summary result.

8. *Fixed effects model:*
   a. *Mantel-Haenszel:* Attempts to derive the most useful summary estimate of effect from the data given in all the studies included in the analysis.
      (1) Similar to analysis of stratified data, where the stratification variable is the individual study.[8]
   b. *Peto:* Utilizes a 2 × 2 table for the observed and expected, and the chi-square value is obtained by $(O_i - E_i)$, and the variance of the expected (V_i) calculated.

9. *Random effects models*
   a. Assumes that the studies that have been included are a representative sample of a hypothetical larger population of studies.
   b. Where there is no heterogeneity between studies, the fixed effect and random effects models yield the same result.
      (1) But where there is heterogeneity, the random effects model may give a substantially different result.
   c. The most widely used random effects model is the DerSimonian-Laird method.
   d. This method weighs the inverse of a combination of within-study variation and between-study variation; because this variance will be larger, the confidence interval of summary measure of effect will be wider.
10. With substantial between-study variance (heterogeneity), the DerSimonian-Laird method gives relatively more weight to the smaller studies.

Table 3-14   Advantages and Disadvantages of Meta-analysis

Advantages
- Utilizes structured research technique to summarize and analyze a body of research studies.
- Represents key study findings (i.e., more differentiated from the conventional review process) that rely on qualitative summaries.
- Capable of finding effects or associations that are obscured in qualitative reviews.
- Provides organized and structured way of handling information from a large number of study findings under review.
- Homogeneity test, which indicates if a grouping of effect sizes are from different studies, shows more variation than would be expected from sampling error alone.
- Capable of performing meta-regression that is not feasible from other types of review.

Disadvantages
- Time consuming and specialized skills.
- Methodological issues—study mixing, different effect sizes, or measure of effect.
- Publication bias.
- Cannot overcome limitations of the individual studies that make up the sample size (k).

XIII. **Study Validity (Bias, Confounding, Random Error) [PHCC.3.6, 3.7]**

A. *Validity* (internal validity) refers to lack of bias and confounding in the design of an epidemiologic study.

B. *External validity* refers to the generalization of the findings from a study to a larger population different from the population that was sampled.[12]

  1. External validity cannot be established without internal validity in the first place.

C. *Bias* is a systematic error that occurs as a result of the investigator's design or conduct of the study that eventually results in inaccurate assessment of the association between the exposure and the outcome of interest.

D. *Types of bias:* (1) recall bias (commonly encountered in case-control study) refers to inability to remember information regarding exposure, especially among the control resulting in misclassification bias; (2) misclassification bias (errors or mistakes in data acquisition that result in wrong grouping of study subjects); (3) information bias (record abstraction, interviewing, surrogate interviews, recall bias, surveillance, reporting); and (4) selection bias.

E. *Surveillance bias:* Because populations with disease are more closely monitored compared with those who do not have the disease, disease ascertainment may be better in the monitored population and may introduce surveillance bias (monitoring of one population [diseased] more than the other [disease-free]). This bias may lead to erroneous estimation of the effect of the disease in the monitored population, thus inflating the point estimate (RR, OR).

F. *Controlling/minimizing bias:* (1) Accurate definition of items, (2) methods of measurement, (3) standardization of procedures, and (4) quality control of data collection and processing.

G. *Confounding:* One of the issues in validation of an epidemiologic research is to assess whether associations between exposure and disease derived from observational epidemiologic studies are of a causal nature or not (due to systematic error, random error, or confounding). Confounding refers to the influence or effect of an extraneous factor(s) on the relationship or associations between

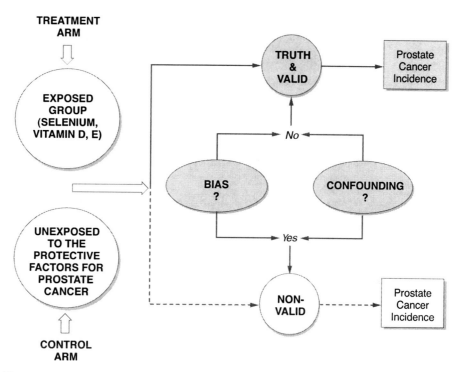

Figure 3-7 Internal Validity—Effect of bias and confounding on validity of a prospective cohort study conducted to determine the effectiveness of selenium, vitamin E and D in reducing prostate cancer incidence.

the exposure and the outcome of interest. Observational studies are potentially subject to the effect of extraneous factors, which may distort the findings of these studies. To be a confounding, the extraneous variable must be (1) a risk factor for the disease being studied and (2) associated with the exposure being studied but is not a consequence of exposure.[13]

1. Occurs when the effects of the exposure are mixed together with the effect of another variable, leading to a bias.

2. If exposure X causes disease Y, Z is a confounder if Z is a known risk factor for disease Y, and Z is associated with X, but Z is not a result of exposure X.

3. *Vignette:* Consider a study to assess the association between coffee drinking (X) and pancreatic cancer risk (Y). The exposure variable is coffee drinking, and coffee drinking is known to be associated with cigarette smoking (Z). Likewise, cigarette smoking is a known risk factor for pancreatic cancer. If

causal association is observed between coffee drinking and pancreatic cancer, this might be due to the confounding effect of smoking. Therefore, to be confounding, smoking must be a risk factor for pancreatic cancer and be associated with coffee drinking.

    a.   If a causal association such as $X \rightarrow Y$ occurs, then this causal relationship may be due to Z (confounder).

H. Confounding per se is not a bias.

I. *Controlling for confounding* is a method of producing an unconfounded effect (point) estimate: (1) During the design phase of the study → (a) restriction, (b) matching, (c) randomization. (2) During analysis phase of the study → (a) restriction, (b) stratification (stratified analysis), (c) multivariable method (analysis).[2,13]

J. Random error refers to unsystematic errors that arise from an unforeseeable and unpredictable process, such as a mistake in assessing the exposure and disease, and sampling variability (unrepresentative sample, or chance).

K. Precision is the lack of random error.

    1. Precision, and hence reduction in random error, may be reduced by (a) increasing the sample size, (b) repeating measurement within a study, and (c) utilizing an efficient study design in order to maximize the amount of information obtained.

    2. Precision (lack of random error) may be influenced by (a) sampling, (b) hypothesis testing and p values, (c) confidence inter-

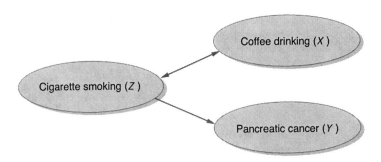

Figure 3-8 Confounding

vals estimation, (d) random variable probability distribution, and (e) sample size and power estimation.[2,6,9]

L. Systematic error may be present in a study despite absence or reduction in random error (study may be precise but findings are inaccurate).

M. *Interaction* is said to occur when the IR of a disease or outcome in the presence of two or more risk factors differs from the IR expected to result from their individual effect. This rate may be greater than what is expected (synergism) or less than what is expected (antagonism).[2,6,9]

N. Like effect measure modifier, interaction is said to occur if there is a difference in the strata-specific risk point estimate (RR, OR) on the basis of the third variable.

O. *Additive model:* occurs in association of effect if the effect of one exposure is added to the effect of the other (e.g., if those with neither exposure have an incidence of 2.0). In those with smoking history, the incidence is 8.0, and 16.0 in those with smoking history and heavy alcohol consumption.[2,8]

   1. The additive model assumes that the incidence will be X in those with both types of risk. What is X? X is 22. Because

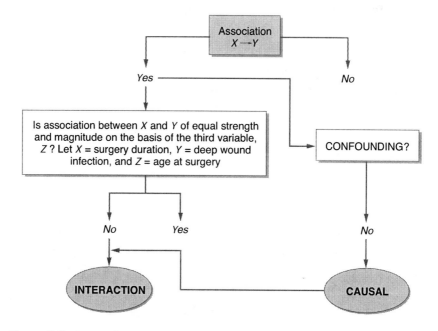

Figure 3-9 Interaction

smoking adds 6.0 to those with no risk, it will be expected to add 6.0 to those with alcohol drinking history.

2. Additive model is not accurate in describing the effect of exposure to two independent factors in disease causation.

P. *Multiplicative model:* appropriate model for describing the effects of two independent factors or exposures in disease causation (e.g., if absence of neither exposure has incidence of 2.0, and those exposed to cigarette smoking have an incidence of 8.0, while those exposed to heavy alcohol consumption have incidence of 16.0).

1. The multiplicative model assumes that the incidence will be Y in those with both risks. What is Y? Y is 64. Because smoking multiplies the risk by four times in the absence of alcohol, we also expect it to multiply the risk in alcohol users by 4 (16×4). If so, the effect of exposure to both smoking and alcohol will be $16 \times 4 = 64$.

Q. Effect measure modifier or effect modification (heterogeneity of effect) refers to the strength of association between exposure and the disease that differs according to level of another variable (effect modifier). For example, age is a modifier in the association between ethnicity and hypertension. Differences are not observed between black and white men under the age of 35 with respect to hypertension incidence. After age 35, incidence tends to be 2 to 3 times higher in blacks relative to whites of the same age.

R. Biologically, an effect measure modifier is the third variable that is not a confounding but enters into a causal pathway between the exposure and the disease of interest.[13] For example, the relationship between lung cancer and cigarette smoking is modified by asbestos, because asbestos exposure has been known to increase the risk of dying by 92 times among smokers, whereas the risk of dying from lung cancer among those exposed to asbestos only is 10-fold. Another example is the modifying effect of cigarette smoking and obesity on the association between oral contraceptives and myocardial infarction in women.

S. Effect measure modifier and confounding: similarities

1. Both confounding and effect measure modifier involve a third variable as well as assessed or evaluated by performing stratified analysis.[9]

T. Effect measure modifier versus confounding:

1. In confounding, one is interested in knowing whether the crude measure of association (unadjusted point estimate) changes (distorted) and whether the stratum-specific and adjusted summary estimate differ from the crude or unadjusted estimate.

BOX 3-7   PROBABILITY VALUE INTERPRETATION & TYPES OF ERRORS

- The p value gives an indication of how plausible the null hypothesis is, but it is not the probability of the null hypothesis being true.
- Simply, the p value is the probability of observing a result as extreme as, or more extreme than, the one actually observed by chance alone; that is, if the null hypothesis is true.
- **TYPE I ERROR**—If one rejects the null hypothesis, and accepts the alternate hypothesis, when in fact the null is TRUE/CORRECT, one commits type I error.
- **TYPE II ERROR**—If one accepts the null hypothesis, implying the rejection of alternate hypothesis, when in fact the alternate hypothesis is TRUE/CORRECT, one commits type II error.

---

2. In effect measure modification, one is interested in finding out if the association differs according to the third variable (the difference in stratum-specific estimate from one another).

U. *Vignette:* Consider a case-control study of the effect of lycopene on CaP stratified by body mass index (BMI) (normal versus overweight). The stratum-specific odds ratio for men with a BMI of $\geq$ 24.99 kg/m^2 = 2.2 and the stratum-specific odds ratio for men with normal BMI ($<$ 24.99 kg/m^2) = 1.0. Does this illustration indicate the presence of effect modifier or confounding by BMI?

V. *Solution:* Because the stratum-specific odds ratio differs between men with normal and abnormal BMI, BMI is an effect measure modifier between lycopene and CaP in men.

1. In this example, the BMI needs to be described or explained in the causal pathway of CaP and does not need to be adjusted for since it is not a confounding.

W. Can the same variable (gender) be an effect measure modifier and confounding in the same setting (simultaneously)?

1. Explore this possibility using the combined odds ratio and stratum specific odds ratio illustration.

XIV. **Epidemiologic Causal Inference [PHCC.3.7, 3.8]**

A. Epidemiologic investigation is concerned with association as well as causal association.

B. Simply, *cause* refers to whatever produces an effect (result, outcome, response variable).

C. Cause may be understood as a factor if its operation increases the frequency of an event (outcome, result).

D. Cause is also described as an event, condition, or characteristic that preceded a health-related event and without which the event would not have occurred at all or would not have occurred until some later time.

E. Causal inference in epidemiology involves two steps: (1) valid result—internal validity of the study (association that is not a result of bias, confounding, and random error) and (2) assessing whether the exposure actually caused the effect (outcome, result).

F. Causal relationship may be:

1. Necessary and sufficient (*necessary* if the outcome occurs only if the causal factor operated and *sufficient* if the operation of the causal factor *always* resulted in the outcome).

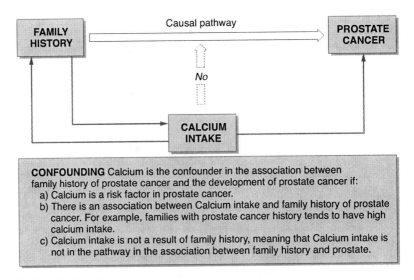

CONFOUNDING Calcium is the confounder in the association between family history of prostate cancer and the development of prostate cancer if:
a) Calcium is a risk factor in prostate cancer.
b) There is an association between Calcium intake and family history of prostate cancer. For example, families with prostate cancer history tends to have high calcium intake.
c) Calcium intake is not a result of family history, meaning that Calcium intake is not in the pathway in the association between family history and prostate.

Figure 3-10 Confounding

2. Necessary but not sufficient.
3. Sufficient but not necessary.
4. Neither sufficient nor necessary, implying that the operation of the causal factor increases the frequency of the causal factor, but the outcome does not always result and the outcome can occur without the operation of the causal factor.[8]

Table 3-15 Bradford Hill's Criteria for Causal Inference	
Criteria	**Explanation**
Temporality	The cause must precede the outcome (disease)
	Complete consensus among investigators and most relevant criterion
	Easily established in prospective studies
Strength of association	Measured by relative risk or odds ratio
	Larger relative risk or odds ratio is more indicative of a stronger association
Dose–response (biologic gradient)	Effect increases as the exposure level increases
Consistency of association	Association is most likely to be causal if observed repeatedly by different persons, in different places, circumstances, and time
Plausibility	Coherency with the current body of knowledge (existence of biologic or social model to explain the association)
Coherence	Cause and effect interpretation of the data should not seriously conflict with generally known facts of the natural history and the biology of the disease
Experiment	If exposure causes a disease, the disease is expected to decline when the exposure is reduced or eliminated
Analogy	Similarities between the observed association and other associations
Specificity	A cause should lead to a single effect and vice versa
	An association is specific when a certain exposure is associated with only one disease

Hill, A.B. The environment and disease: Association or causation? *Proc R Soc Med.* 1965; 58:295–300.

G. *Rothman's notion of causality: component cause model (causal pies)*
   [PHCC.3.7]
   1. *Sufficient cause:* complete causal mechanism that inevitably
      produces disease.
   2. *Component cause:* each participating factor in a sufficient cause.
   3. *Necessary cause:* a causal component that is a member of
      every sufficient cause.
   4. The causal pies model indicates that a sufficient cause is not a
      single factor but rather a minimal set of factors that unavoidably
      produce disease, implying that the termination of the action of a
      single causal component blocks the completion of a sufficient
      cause, thus preventing disease occurrence by that pathway.[14]

H. *Vignette 1:* Consider an epidemiologic investigation conducted to
   assess the association between exposure to sulfur and brain
   tumor in children. If the investigator wishes to compare the findings in this study with other evidence, which criteria according
   to Bradford Hill might be worth considering, and what sort of
   study design may provide a more valid and reliable comparison?
   1. *Solution:* Evidence from one study may be compared with
      another in terms of Hill's criteria of consistency, plausibility,
      coherence, and specificity. The design most appropriate will
      be prospective studies.

I. *Vignette 2:* Consider an investigator who wishes to examine published studies on the evidence of estrogen replacement therapy in
   post-menopausal breast cancer. If he wishes to examine the features consistent with causation using Bradford Hill criteria, which
   features should be taken into consideration?
   1. *Solution:* Bradford Hill's features consistent with causation are
      (a) temporal sequence, (b) strength of association, (c) dose
      response, (d) consistency, and (e) specificity.

J. *Vignette 3:* Consider an investigation of epidemiologic causal
   inference that attempts to examine the study validity prior to
   assessing whether the exposure actually led to the disease. Which
   aspects of the study must he or she consider in order to determine if the observed result was valid?
   1. *Solution:* The first step in epidemiologic causal inference is to
      illustrate that the result was not due to (a) systematic error
      (bias), (b) confounding, or (c) random error.

XV. Disease Screening: Principles, Advantages, and Limitations

   A. Population screening refers to early screening and treatment in large groups in order to reduce morbidity or mortality from the specified disease among the screened.

   B. Screening for the purpose of disease control or mortality reduction involves the examination of asymptomatic or preclinical cases for the purpose of correctly classifying the diseased as positive and nondiseased as negative.[2,14,15]

   C. *Diagnostic or screening test accuracy/validity:* refers to the ability of the test to accurately distinguish those who do and do not have a specific disease.[16] Sensitivity and specificity are traditionally used to determine the validity of a diagnostic test. *Sensitivity:* the ability of the test to classify correctly those who have the disease or specific/targeted disorder. Sensitivity is represented by $a / (a + c)$ in a 2×2 contingent table. "SnNout" is used to describe sensitivity, meaning that when "sen"sitivity is high, a "n"egative result rules "out" diagnosis.

   D. *Specificity:* the ability of the test to classify correctly those without the disease as nondiseased. Specificity is represented by $d / (b + d)$. "SpPin," which is used to describe specificity, implies that a very high specificity with a positive result effectively rules in the diagnosis.

   E. Predictive value of the test addresses the effectiveness of the test to accurately identify those with the disease and those without.

   F. The positive predictive value of the test addresses the question: If the test result is positive in an individual, what is the probability that such individual has the disease? This is estimated by: $a / (a + b)$.

   G. The negative predictive value addresses the probability of an individual with a negative test to be disease-free. This is estimated by $d / (c + d)$.

   H. False positive error rate is estimated by $1 -$ specificity $= b / (b + d)$.

   I. False negative error rate is estimated by $1 -$ sensitivity $= c / (a + c)$.

   J. Prevalence $= (a + c) / (a + b + c + d)$.

   K. LR+, which is the likelihood ratio for a positive test is estimated by Sensitivity $/ (1 -$ specificity).

   L. LR−, which is the likelihood ratio for a negative test is estimated by $(1 -$ Sensitivity$) /$ Specificity.

M. Post-test probability is estimated by Post-test odds / (Post-test odds + 1), where pre-test odds is estimated by Prevalence / (1 − Prevalence) and post-test odds is estimated by Pre-test odds × Likelihood ratio.

BOX 3-8   DIAGNOSTIC/SCREENING TEST-FALSE POSITIVE ERROR RATE
- False positive error rate (alpha error rate or type I error rate) simply referring to error committed by asserting that a proposition is TRUE, when it is indeed NOT TRUE (FALSE).
- If a test is not SPECIFIC, this will lead to the test to falsely indicate the presence of a disease in non-disease subjects.
- The rate upon which this occurs is termed, false positive error rate, and is mathematically given by: $B / (B + D)$.
- False positive error rate is related to specificity: FP(rate) + Specificity = 1.0 (100%).

N. *Vignette:* Consider a population of 2,000 people, of whom 200 have unicameral bone cysts and 1,800 do not. If 160 with the disease were correctly identified as positive by the test, 40 were not. Of the 1,800 who did not have the disease, 1,600 were correctly classified as negative. Calculate (1) sensitivity, (2) specificity, (3) positive predictive value, and (4) negative predictive value.
  1. *Solution:* (a) Sensitivity = $a / (a + c)$; substituting: 160 ÷ 200 = 80%; (b) Specificity = $d / (d + b)$ = 1,600 ÷ 1,800 = 89%; (c) Positive predictive value = $a / (a + b)$ = 160 ÷ 360 = 44.4%; and (d) Negative predictive value = $d / (c + d)$ = 1,600 ÷ 1,640 = 97.6%.

Table 3-16   A 2 × 2 Contingency Table Illustrating Diagnostic Test Results

Test Result	Population (Target)	
	Disease	Nondisease or Disease-free
Positive	a	b
Negative	c	d

Abbreviation: a = true-positive, b = false-positive, c = false-negative and d = true-negative.

Sensitivity = $a / (a + c)$; Specificity = $d / (b + d)$; Positive predictive value (PPV) = $a / (a + b)$; Negative predictive value = $d / (c + d)$; False-positive rate = $c / (a + c)$; False-negative rate = $b / (b + d)$.

O. *Relationship between disease prevalence and predictive value:* the higher the prevalence in the population at risk or screened population, the higher the positive predictive value.

P. *Advantage of screening:* screening is most productive and efficient if it is directed at a high-risk population.

Q. Screening of high-risk population may motivate participants who may follow recommendation after the screening and seek medical services given positive test results.

R. *Disadvantage of screening:* If the entire population is screened and the condition is infrequent (low prevalence), this will imply wasteful resources, yielding few undetected cases compared to the effort invested in the screening.

S. *Issues in early disease detection:* What are the benefits of screening?

   1. *Early disease detection:* The natural history of disease involves (a) a *preclinical phase,* which is the phase that may be termed the biological or psychological onset, but the symptoms have not yet occurred; (b) a *clinical phase,* which is the period after which the symptoms occurred; (c) a *detectable preclinical phase,* whish is the natural stage of the disease where the disease is detected by screening; (d) *lead time,* which is the interval by which the time of diagnosis is advanced by screening and early detection of disease relative to the usual time of diagnosis; and (e) a *critical point,* which refers to a point in the natural history of the disease in which the condition is potentially curable, implying optimal treatment potential.

   2. Inability to identify a critical point in natural history of disease, screening, and early detection questions the benefit of screening.

   3. Effectiveness of screening includes (a) mortality reduction in the high-risk population screened, (b) reduction in case fatality, (c) increase in the percent of asymptomatic cases, (d) minimized complications, (e) reduction in recurrent cases or malignancies, and (f) improvement in the quality of life.[2,17]

T. Issues in screening include: (1) sensitivity and specificity of the screening test as well as the predictive values, (2) false-positive test results, (3) cost of early detection, (4) emotional and physical adverse effects of screening, and (5) benefit of the screening.[2,18]

BOX 3-9   RELIABILITY TEST: KAPPA STATISTIC

- Reliability studies are designed to quantify the reproducibility of the same variable, for example, daily dietary intake of a particular food, measured more than once.
- Kappa, which is a measure of agreement "beyond chance," is used as a measure reproducibility between repeated assessments of the same variable.
- The chi-square test of association between the two surveys responses, though performable, will not give a quantitative measure of the reproducibility between the responses at the two surveys.
- Using Kappa statistics (κ), is the appropriate test to measure reproducibility: Po $-$ Pe / 1 $-$ Pe, where Po is the observed probability of the concordance between two surveys, and Pe is the expected probability of concordance between the two surveys.
- Kappa is interpreted as, $\kappa > 0.75$ (75%) indicates excellent reproducibility, 0.4 (40%) $\leq \kappa \leq 0.75$ (75%), good reproducibility while $0 \leq \kappa < 0.4$ (40%) denotes marginal/poor reproducibility. $+1.0$ is indicative of a perfect agreement, while 0.0 indicates a complete independent between the two surveys.
- Specificity and sensitivity would be more appropriate indices of reliability or reproducibility if the investigators were interested in the concordance between responses on two different variables, where one of the variables is considered to be the cold standard.

U. *Biases in disease screening and detection:* (1) referral bias, also referred to as volunteer bias; (2) length-biased sampling associated with prognostic selection. This bias refers to a selection bias in which screening involves the selection of cases of disease with better prognosis.[2,9] (3) lead time bias; and (4) overdiagnosis bias. Other biases in disease screening and detection include:

   1. Lead time bias refers to the apparent increase in survival time after diagnosis resulting from earlier time of diagnosis rather than later time of death.
   2. Length bias refer to the tendency, in a population screening effort, to detect preferentially the longer, more indolent cases of any particular disease.

V. *Vignette:* Consider a new screening program for CaP in County X. The CaP screening program used a test that is effective in screening for early stage CaP. Assume that there is no effective treatment for CaP and, as such, the screening results do not change in the natural history or course of CaP. Second, assume that the rates observed are based on all known cases of CaP, and that there are no changes in the quality of death certification for CaP. With these assumptions, (1) what will be the influence of this screening test on incidence and prevalence proportion during the first year of this program? (2) What will be the influence of this screening on case-fatality and mortality rate of CaP during the first year of CaP screening?

1. *Solutions:* (a) There will be an increase in both incidence rate and prevalence proportion. (b) There will be a decrease in case-fatality rate, while the mortality rate will remain constant due to the assumption that changes had not been observed with respect to the quality of death certification.

XVI. **Ethical and Legal Duties of Epidemiology in Study Design, Data Collection, Analysis, and Dissemination of Study Findings**

A. All scientific work is incomplete, whether it be observational or experimental. Also, all scientific work is liable to be upset or modified by advancing knowledge.[19]

B. Epidemiology is largely an observational science and therefore incomplete and subject to modification as new data become available.

C. Whereas the goal of epidemiology is not to prevent and control diseases, epidemiology plays a major role in providing scientific and relevant data for the development of policies that affect human health.

D. Epidemiologic knowledge is used to design intervention in order to control disease and promote the health of the community and public as well as inform clinical medicine in terms of its application in individual cases (clinical epidemiology).

E. *Ethical considerations:* Epidemiologic designs including clinical trials must be ethically feasible involving informed consent prior to subjects' recruitments; observation of moral principles in terms of data collection, safety, and monitoring; and they must discourage, at all times, the misuse of data. Epidemiologic ethical decisions must be driven by *primum non nocere,* meaning, "first do no harm"—physical or mental—and implying adherence to nonmaleficence principles in study designs, conduct, and interpretation.

1. The analysis of epidemiologic data must be guided by ethical principles of trust, truthfulness, confidentiality, and privacy.

2. The findings from epidemiologic data must be objective and driven by the facts as revealed in the data and not subjective imposition of findings that are not supported by data.

3. Epidemiologic data analysis must encourage independent analysis for result validation, verification, and replication. Publications and authorship must be based on individual contributions to the study without influence of pseudo-authors or individuals paid to place their names on the authorship who made no contributions to the paper.

4. Conflict of interest may generate actual or perceived bias and should be avoided in all epidemiologic designs and interpretations.

F. *Legal considerations:* Legislation and governmental social control involves public policy, which implies the role of epidemiology in informing policies on health risk.

G. Policy decision regarding risk considers epidemiologic findings based on sound study designs, consideration of bias, confounding, and effect measure modifiers in the communication of the results.[2,20]

H. Epidemiology plays an important role in the objective interpretation of study findings regarding the risk of exposure or benefits of intervention or treatment for health policy development.

I. In the procedural justice arena, epidemiology provides the data necessary for the legal system to arrive at a decision or settlement regarding culpability and legal responsibilities (torts litigation) of corporations, such as energy and drug companies, in regard to exposure to occupational hazards, toxic substances that may later predispose to tumors, malignancies, chronic diseases, and early mortality.

J. The use of epidemiologic evidence in the judiciary system will increase as epidemiologic evidence relies more and more on molecular epidemiologic designs and interpretation, which implies the penetration of the epidemiologic black box to uncover gene-environment and molecular basis of exposure-induced diseases.

REFERENCES

1. Last JM. *A Dictionary of Epidemiology*. 3rd ed. New York: Oxford University Press; 1995.
2. Gordis, L. *Epidemiology*. 3rd ed. Philadelphia: Elsevier Saunders; 2004.
3. Savitz DA. *Interpreting Epidemiologic Evidence*. New York: Oxford University Press; 2003.
4. Mausner J, Kramer S. *Epidemiology—An Introductory Text*. 2nd ed. Philadelphia: Saunders; 1985.
5. MacMahan B, Trichopoulos D. *Epidemiology, Principles & Methods*. 2nd ed. Boston: Little, Brown & Company; 1996.
6. Rothman KJ. *Epidemiology, An Introduction*. New York: Oxford University Press; 2002.
7. Hennekens CH, Buring JE. *Epidemiology in Medicine*. Boston: Little Brown & Company; 1987.
8. Elwood M. *Critical Appraisal of Epidemiological Studies in Clinical Trials*. 2nd ed. New York: Oxford University Press; 2003.
9. Aschengrau A, Seage III GR. *Essentials of Epidemiology*. Sudbury, MA: Jones and Bartlett; 2003.
10. Friis RH, Sellers TA. *Epidemiology for Public Health Practice*. Frederick, MD: Aspen Publications; 1996.
11. Lipsey MW, Wilson D. *Practical Meta-analysis*. Thousand Oaks, CA: Sage Publications; 2001.
12. Szklo M, Nieto J. *Epidemiology: Beyond the Basics*. Sudbury, MA: Jones and Bartlett; 2003.
13. Schlesselman JJ. *Case-Control Studies. Design, Conduct, Analysis*. New York: Oxford University Press; 1982.
14. Rothman KJ. *Modern Epidemiology*. Boston: Little, Brown & Company; 1986.
15. Jekel JF, Katz DL, Elmore JG. *Epidemiology, Biostatistics, and Preventive Medicine*. Philadelphia: Saunders; 2001.
16. Katz DL. *Clinical Epidemiology & Evidence-Based Medicine: Fundamental Principles of Clinical Reasoning & Research*. Thousand Oaks, CA: Sage; 2001.
17. Dawson-Saunders B, Trap RG. *Basic and Clinical Biostatistics*. 2nd ed. Norwalk, CT: Appleton & Lange; 1994.
18. Garb JL. *Understanding Medical Research: A Practitioner's Guide*. Boston: Little, Brown & Company; 2000.
19. Bradford Hill, President's Address, Royal Society of Medicine, 1965.
20. Taubes G. Epidemiology faces its limits. *Science*. 1995;269:164–169.

Chapter 4

Health Policy and Management Sciences in Public Health

Larry Holmes, Jr., Doriel D. Ward, Gbadebo Ogungbade, and Joan Nwuli

HEALTH POLICY AND MANAGEMENT SCIENCES CORE COMPETENCIES LEARNING OBJECTIVES

Health policy and management is a multidisciplinary field of inquiry and practice concerned with the delivery, quality, and costs of health care for individuals and populations. This definition assumes both a managerial and a policy concern with the structure, process, and outcomes of health services, including the costs, financing, organization, outcomes, and accessibility of care.

PHCC.4.1. Identify the main components and issues of the organization, financing, and delivery of health services and public health systems in the United States.

PHCC.4.2. Discuss the policy process for improving the health status of populations.

PHCC.4.3. Describe the legal and ethical bases for public health and health services.

PHCC.4.4. Apply quality and performance improvement concepts to address organizational performance issues.

PHCC.4.5. Demonstrate leadership skills for building partnerships.

PHCC.4.6. Apply principles of strategic planning and marketing to public health.

PHCC.4.7. Communicate health policy and management issues using appropriate channels and technologies.

PHCC.4.8.	Apply the principles of program planning, development, budgeting, management, and evaluation in organizational and community initiatives.
PHCC.4.9.	Explain methods of ensuring community health safety and preparedness.
PHCC.4.10.	Apply "systems thinking" for resolving organizational problems.

PREVIEW

Management and policy sciences (MAPS) encompass the core disciplines of public health and play a significant role in the policy development and assurance of public health services. MAPS is a multidisciplinary field of inquiry and practice concerned with the delivery, quality, and costs of health care for individuals and populations. This description of MAPS assumes both a managerial and a policy concern with the structure, process, and outcomes of health services, including the costs, financing, organization, outcomes, and accessibility of care.

This chapter presents the role of policy in public health services implementation and intervention designs to control diseases and promote health, the governmental role in health policy development, the substance of public health law, and the public health federal regulations, with an emphasis on the Health Insurance Portability and Accountability Act (HIPAA). Public health ethics is presented in contrast to medical ethics, focusing mainly on human subjects in research as well as the elements of informed consent. Equity in health is presented in terms of the inequality in the provision of quality care due to personal characteristics such as race/ethnicity, gender, socioeconomic status, and age, with stress on the health effects of insurance coverage and racial/ethnic disparities. The role of public health in disaster preparedness is presented, with the intent to illustrate the essentials of data gathered from public health assessment in preparing for future disaster. The quality and performance improvement are presented as well as strategic planning and marketing. These two aspects emphasize the role of strategic planning and accountability in the delivery of public health services. Like in most organizations, conflict resolution is essential in maintaining the continued existence of organization or industry. The theories applicable to public health in this vein are discussed, mainly "systems thinking" and its application to public health issues. Finally, program development, evaluation, and reporting are presented with a logic model to indicate the nonlinearity of program development, implementation, and evaluation.

I.   **Management and Policy Sciences and Public Health**
   A. Policy development, organization, and management of public health services are essential functions of public health.
      [PHCC.4.2] *Policy* refers to the process by which governments, institutions, or organizations translate their political vision into programs and actions to deliver "outcomes," or desired changes in the real world.[1] *Health policy* can be conceived as a single statement or a set of laws, regulations, or, more vaguely, guiding principles formulated to manage a particular health issue or to resolve more fundamental problems. Health policy thus represents an action plan that steers the direction of a social, professional, and often government response to a health-related issue. The health policy makers attempt to find a way among competing economic, political, value-based, and social needs, to mention the obvious, in order to define compromise actions that can be taken in practice.[2]
   B. Policy development as a core function of public health involves:
      1. Broad community involvement.
      2. Promotion of the scientific basis of decision making.
      3. Strategic approach.
      4. Development of comprehensive public health policies.[3]
   C. Policy development serves as a core function of public health. Policy can improve health by initiating transition in physical, economic, and social environments. The implementation of public health services requires policy development and planning or management:
      1. Systematic communitywide planning for health improvement.
      2. Developing and tracking measurable objectives.
      3. Developing policy and legislation to the practice of public health.

4. Implementing joint evaluation with the medical care system.
5. Leadership development at all levels.[3,4]

D. Framework for examining public health system performance [PHCC.4.1]

1. The framework for examining public health system performance involves capacity, process, and outcomes.
2. The *capacity* level refers to the inputs that involve interaction with workforce, information, organization, relationship, facilities, and funding.
3. The *process* that is the essential public health services refers to the core functions of public health: assessment, policy development, and assurance.
4. The *outcome* refers to the output (program and services consistent with mandates, community needs, and priorities) that leads to the outcomes (improved organizational performance and improved program performance).[4–6]

II. **Basics of Policy Formulation and Implementation [PHCC.4.2]**

A. If public health is to meet its substance of disease control and health promotions, it must rely on evidence-based policies.
B. The use of evidence-based policy and practice can effectively lead to improvement in the health of the population.
C. The movement for evidence-based policy and practice and for the use of research evidence in the work of the professions started in medicine in the early 1990s.

1. It has grown in influence and spread across a number of other fields.
2. It is necessary in order to track performance and ensure accountability.[7,8]

D. Building on a tradition of evidence-based medicine, this approach is receiving increasing attention in new fields of professional practice such as education, social work, criminal justice, and others.
E. The process of sourcing the evidence must be incorporated as an integral part of the policy formulation itself.[2,4,9]
F. The effectiveness of this approach is also based on the integrity of the processes of sourcing the evidence, interpreting the informa-

tion, utilizing the knowledge, understanding and adopting the evidence, evaluating and adapting it, and applying and acting on it.[7,9]

  G. The overall process for the evidence-based policy formulation is illustrated by:

    1. The policy idea.

    2. Sourcing the evidence, that is, implying knowledge, research, ideas/interests, politics, and economics.

    3. Evidence usage.

    4. Consideration of the capacity to implement.[8–10]

  H. *Stages in policy development*

    1. Problem identification.

    2. Priority setting.

    3. Policy formulation and design.

    4. Passage of policy instruments.

    5. Implementation.

    6. Evaluation.[7–9]

  I. *Tools and resources to support policy development*

    1. Data gathering and analysis.[2]

    2. Research effectiveness of strategies.

    3. Media strategies (in collaboration with the communications coordinator).

    4. Training.[2]

    5. Evaluation.

III. Health Policies and the Governmental Role in Development and Implementation [PHCC.4.1, 4.2, 4.7]

  A. Health policy involves all sectors of the government:

    1. *Federal*

      a. U.S. Department of Health and Human Services

        (1) Agencies include the National Institutes of Health (NIH), the Centers for Disease Control and Prevention, the U.S. Food and Drug Administration, the Agency for Healthcare Research and Quality, etc.

        (2) Programs include Medicare, Medicaid, State Children's Health Insurance Program (SCHIP), Maternal and Child Health (MCH), and family planning.

BOX 4-1   SELECTED AGENCIES, PUBLIC AND PRIVATE SECTORS, AND LEVEL OF INVOLVEMENTS IN PUBLIC HEALTH SERVICES

- The CDC focuses on crisis-oriented infectious diseases, such as anthrax diagnosed in postal workers.
- The NIH focuses on basic sciences research aimed at curing human diseases, such as investigating the use of statin drugs to reduce the incidence of Alzheimer's disease.
- The Bill and Melinda Gates Foundation primarily focuses on improving global health diseases, such as HIV, malaria, and tuberculosis.
- State health departments hold the primary constitutional authority to address policies concerning improvement of birth outcomes, including birth weight, preterm births, and infant mortality and morbidity.
- Local health departments (county and city) focus on day-to-day operations of public health clinics.

---

    2. *State*
        a. Departments of health, human services, or social services.
        b. Divisions of insurance.
        c. Medical schools and affiliated teaching hospitals.
    3. *Local*
        a. Departments of public health.
  B. *Spending on health:*
    1. Accounts for a sizable share of state spending; half from federal funds.
    2. Total U.S. state health spending in the years 2002–2003 accounted for $1.1 trillion.[11]
  C. *States' role in health policy*
    1. *Regulator*
        a. Health professional licensing.
        b. Health facilities licensing.
        c. Regulations for insurance companies and managed care organizations.
    2. *Purchaser*
        a. Medicaid beneficiaries.
        b. SCHIP.
        c. State employees and retirees.

3. State health spending is dominated by Medicaid.[11]
   a. Medicaid is administered by the states, with federal over-sight and shared federal/state financing (57% federal).
   b. Medicaid provides health and long-term care services for more than 52 million low-income people.
      (1) 39 million adults and children in low-income families.
      (2) 13 million frail elders and people with disabilities, including more than 6 million Medicare beneficiaries.
4. Pays for nearly 1 in 5 healthcare dollars and 1 in 2 nursing home dollars.
5. Large variation across states in eligibility and scope of benefits.
6. *Provider*
   a. Facilities for the developmentally disabled and mental health hospitals.
   b. State-operated nursing homes and veterans' homes.
   c. Medical schools and affiliated teaching hospitals.
   d. *Prisons:*
      (1) States spent $4.0 billion on inmate medical care in 2003.[11]
      (2) Increase in spending as a result of larger prison popula-tion, increase in HIV/AIDS, and aging of prison population.
   e. Public and population health.
   f. Programs for targeted populations.
D. *Public health functions of the state* [PHCC.4.1]
   1. Vital statistics records and reporting.
   2. Disease surveillance.
   3. Injury prevention and public safety.
   4. Staff and operate pathology lab.
   5. Medical research.
   6. Protection against environmental hazards.
E. *Specific services provided by the state*
   1. Title V.
   2. MCH Program.
   3. Drug assistance for seniors.
   4. Chronic disease hospitals and programs.
   5. Hearing aid assistance.
   6. Adult day care for persons with Alzheimer's disease.

7. Health grants.
8. Medically handicapped children.
9. Women, Infants, and Children programs.
10. Pregnancy outreach and counseling.
11. Chronic renal disease treatment programs.
12. AIDS treatment.
13. Breast and cervical cancer screening and treatment.
14. Tuberculosis programs.
15. Emergency health services.
16. Adult genetics programs.
17. Phenylketonuria testing.

F. *Congress and health policy* [**PHCC.4.3**]
  1. Congress plays a major role in development of health policy.[12]
     a. Medicare.
     b. Medicaid.
     c. NIH.
     d. Health policy is a bipartisan priority.
     e. Authority spread across several committees.
     f. Involvement includes regulatory, programmatic, financing, and oversight.
  2. *Top three health care priorities for the U.S. Congress, 2005:*[12]
     a. Lowering cost of health care and insurance—63%.
     b. Increasing number of Americans without insurance—57%.
     c. Improving nation's ability to respond to bioterrorism—50%.
  3. *Congressional legislation on health care (illustrative legislations):*
     a. Enactment of Medicare and Medicaid (1965).
     b. Employee Retirement Income Security Act (ERISA) (1974).
     c. Americans with Disabilities Act (1990).
     d. Family Medical Leave Act (1993).
     e. Temporary Assistance for Needy Families (TANF) (1996).
     f. HIPAA (1996).
     g. SCHIP (1997).
     h. Medicare Modernization Act (2003).
  4. *Senate Health, Education, Labor, and Pensions (HELP) Committee*—chief health responsibilities:
     a. Aging policy.
     b. Biomedical research and development.
     c. Domestic activities of the American National Red Cross.

       d. Individuals with disabilities.

       e. Occupational safety and health, including the welfare of miners.

       f. Public health.

  5. *House Committee on Energy and Commerce*—chief health responsibilities:

       a. Medicaid.

       b. Medicare.

       c. Public health programs.

       d. Food and drug safety.

       e. Hospital construction, mental health and research, biomedical programs, and health protection in general.

  6. *House Committee on Ways and Means*—chief health responsibilities:

       a. Government payments for programs in Social Security Act: Medicare, welfare (TANF), Supplemental Security Income (SSI), Social Services (Title XX).

       b. Tax credits and related matters in Tax Code dealing with health insurance premiums.

  7. *House Committee on Finance*—chief health responsibilities:

       a. Health programs under the Social Security Act and health programs financed by a specific tax or trust fund, including Medicaid, Medicare, SCHIP, welfare (TANF), MCH block grant, SSI, ERISA (with HELP Committee).

       b. Revenue measures generally, except as provided in the Congressional Budget Act of 1974.[12]

IV. Public Health Laws and Application to Health Promotion and Disease Prevention [PHCC.4.3]

  A. Constitutional right to privacy: *Whalen v. Roe* grants limited right to health information privacy.

  B. Privacy is inherent in U.S. history and the Constitution.

    1. Federal law

       a. Privacy Act of 1974.

       b. HIPAA privacy rules.

    2. State law

       a. Disease specific.

       b. Extra confidentiality for certain conditions.

    3. Tort

C. Public Law 104-191: Health Insurance Portability and Accountability Act of 1996 [13-16]
   1. *Electronic transactions and code sets*[13,16]
      a. Standardizes the data content and format of 10 financial or administrative transactions related to health care (e.g., claims, payments).
      b. Standardizes medical codes (no local codes, e.g., "Y" codes).
   2. *Privacy of Individually Identifiable Health Information*
      a. Regulates uses and disclosures of individually identifiable health information.
      b. Provides patient rights with respect to their health information.
      c. Establishes requirements to ensure privacy of patient.
   3. *HIPAA-covered entities*
      a. *Health plans*
         (1) Provides or pays for the cost of healthcare services.
         (2) Includes Medicaid, Medicare, HealthChoice, Veterans Health Program, Military Health Plan, Indian Health Service, and others.
         (3) Excludes most other government-funded programs.
      b. Healthcare providers who conduct any of the HIPAA-regulated transactions electronically.
      c. Healthcare clearinghouses (not applicable to Division of Public Health).
D. *Privacy regulation*[13,14]
   1. The privacy regulation establishes a federal floor of safeguards to protect the confidentiality of health information.
   2. Applies to Protected Health Information (PHI), which is:
      a. Individually identifiable health information.
      b. Transmitted or maintained in any form or medium (electronic, written, oral).
   3. PHI is any information, including demographic information, collected from an individual that:
      a. Is created or received by a healthcare provider, health plan, employer, or healthcare clearinghouse.
      b. Relates to the past, present, or future physical or mental health or condition of an individual; the provision of health care to an individual; or the past, present, or future payment of the provision of health care to an individual.

E. *HIPAA: Individual rights*[15,16]
  1. Right to be informed of protections on and use of their health information through a notice of privacy practices.
  2. Right to inspect, copy, and review their records.
  3. Right to request amendments to their records.
  4. Right to request restrictions on use and disclosure of health information.
  5. Right to request reasonable personal communications.
  6. Right to an accounting of disclosures of their health information.
  7. Right to file a complaint against covered entity.

V. **Public Health Ethics [PHCC.4.3]**
  A. Ethical values include[17–20]
    1. Respect for persons or autonomy.
    2. Trusting relationships.
    3. Economic harms.
  B. Medical ethics is primarily concerned with patient–provider relationships or interactions.
  C. Public health ethics is concerned with institutions and populations.
    1. The foci of medical ethics are autonomy, goodness, and beneficence.
    2. Public health ethics focuses on interdependence, participation, and scientific information.
  D. *Human subjects in research*
    1. *Nuremberg Code (Human Experimentation):* The voluntary consent of the human subject is absolutely essential. This means that the person involved should have legal capacity to give consent; should be so situated as to be able to exercise free power of choice, without the intervention of any element of force, fraud, deceit, duress, overreaching, or other ulterior form of constraint or coercion; and should have sufficient knowledge and comprehension of the elements of the subject matter involved as to enable him or her to make an informed and enlightened decision. This latter element requires that before the acceptance of an affirmative decision by the experimental subject, there should be made known to him or her the nature, duration, and purpose of the experiment; the method and means by which it is to be conducted; all inconveniences and hazards to be reasonably expected; and the

effects upon his or her health or person that may possibly come from his or her participation in the experiment.[17]

2. The duty and responsibility for ascertaining the quality of the consent rests upon each individual who initiates, directs, or engages in the experiment. It is a personal duty and responsibility that may not be delegated to another with impunity.

3. Title 45 (Public Welfare Department of Health and Human Services), Part 46 (Protection of Human Subjects), of the Code of Federal Regulations sets the guidelines for the protection of human subjects in research.[17]

4. *Belmont Report on Human Subject Protection (National Commission for the Protection of Human Subjects of Biomedical and Behavioral Research):* One of the charges to the Commission was to identify the basic ethical principles that should underlie the conduct of biomedical and behavioral research involving human subjects and to develop guidelines that should be followed to ensure that such research is conducted in accordance with those principles. In carrying out these principles, the Commission was directed to consider:

    a. The boundaries between biomedical and behavioral research and the accepted and routine practice of medicine.

    b. The role of assessment of risk-benefit criteria in the determination of the appropriateness of research involving human subjects.

    c. Appropriate guidelines for the selection of human subjects for participation in such research.

    d. The nature and definition of informed consent in various research settings.

5. *World Medical Association Declaration of Helsinki: Ethical Principles for Medical Research Involving Human Subjects*[19]

    a. The World Medical Association has developed the Declaration of Helsinki as a statement of ethical principles to provide guidance to physicians and other participants in medical research involving human subjects.

    b. Medical research involving human subjects includes research on identifiable human material or identifiable data.

    c. It is the duty of the physician to promote and safeguard the health of the people. The physician's knowledge and conscience are dedicated to the fulfillment of this duty.

    d. The Declaration of Geneva of the World Medical Association binds the physician with the words, "The health of my patient will be my first consideration," and the International Code of Medical Ethics declares that, "A physician shall act only in the patient's interest when providing medical care which might have the effect of weakening the physical and mental condition of the patient."

VI. **Health Disparities: Insurance and Race/Ethnicity [PHCC.4.3, 4.5, 4.7]**

  A. Health insurance and population health.

  B. Most Americans have health insurance, but millions do not; many who are well covered today may find themselves uninsured or underinsured in the future.[21]

  C. Studies have persistently shown the nexus between disease prognosis and mortality and insurance coverage.

  D. Without good insurance coverage, people simply do not get the care they need, when they need it.

  E. There are differences between insured and uninsured regarding barriers to health care.

Table 4-1 Differences Between Insured and Uninsured with Respect to Obstacles to Receiving Health Care

Obstacles to Health Care	Uninsured (%)	Insured (Public and Private) (%)
Postpone seeking care because of cost	47	15
Need care but did not get it	35	9
Did not fill a prescription because of cost	37	13
Had problems paying medical bills	36	16
Contacted by collection agency about medical bills	23	8

Source: Kaiser 2003 Health Insurance Survey.

F. *Health risk—uninsured versus insured*
1. Uninsured people, compared with those privately insured, are less likely to be diagnosed with early onset tumor (prostate, breast, melanoma, colorectal cancer) and are more likely to be diagnosed with late onset malignancy.
2. People in poor health are twice as likely to have a lengthy spell without coverage.

G. *Insurance distribution*[21,22–24]
1. At age 65, most people in the United States qualify for Medicare.
2. Before age 65, we rely on various sources of coverage.
3. About 15% of the nonelderly are covered under public programs—mostly Medicaid, which is a safety net program for certain low-income people: children, parents of dependent children, pregnant women, and people with disabilities who cannot work.
4. The vast majority of people under age 65 rely on private health insurance.
5. The $1.9 trillion healthcare system in 2004 indicated that more than one-third of total healthcare spending was financed by private health insurance.
6. More than 60% of the nonelderly get private health insurance at work, as a benefit from their own job or as the spouse or dependent of a working family member.
7. About 5% of the nonelderly buy health insurance on their own in what is called the "individual insurance market."
8. The rest—18% or almost 46 million nonelderly Americans—are uninsured.

H. *Private insurance model*
1. Indemnity.
2. "Managed care"
    a. Preferred provider organization.
    b. Health maintenance organization.
    c. Point of service.
3. "Consumer-directed" health arrangements.
4. Most people with private insurance have some form of managed care, implying that coverage is most comprehensive when the physician is seen in a specified network. Care provided out of network may not be covered, or the policyholder

may be required to pay more out of pocket. Different models vary in specifics of network policies, how they are financed, access to specialists, benefits, and cost-sharing.

5. Consumer-directed health plans are characterized by high cost-sharing and represent a fundamental shift, whereby the consumer is responsible for more of the purchasing of health-care plans.

I. *Health insurance dynamics*

1. There are 45 million uninsured in a 1-year snapshot, but 80 million people may lack coverage for at least 1 month over a 2-year period.

2. Coverage options can change with:
   a. Loss or change of job.
   b. Change in family status (e.g., divorce, death of spouse).
   c. Birthday (e.g., 19th).
   d. Relocation—moving.
   e. Change in health status.

3. Similarly, the snapshot shows 5% in the individual market, but one in four adults will try to buy individual coverage during a 3-year period.

4. On average, 2 million Americans lose or change coverage every month.

5. Of these 2 million people, most will be uninsured for at least 30 days, then obtain new coverage. However, for some it will take a year or longer before they regain insurance.

J. *Insurance eligibility: Employer-sponsored insurance* is less likely to be offered to:

1. Employees of small relative to large firms.
2. Part-time/seasonal workers compared to full-time.
3. Low-wage workers.
4. Newly hired workers (waiting periods).
5. Dependents relative to employees.
6. Retirees.

K. Eligibility is not based on health status.

L. *Individual insurance*

1. Purchased by individuals.
2. Age and health status are a determining factor (medical underwriting).

M. *Health conditions determining individual insurance:* Individual insurance may be denied due to the following health conditions:

1. *Always denied*
   a. Cancer.
   b. Multiple sclerosis.
   c. HIV/AIDS.
   d. Pregnancy.
   e. Diabetes.
   f. Stroke.

2. *Often denied*
   a. Overweight.
   b. High blood pressure.
   c. Cancer history.
   d. Asthma.

3. *Sometimes denied*
   a. Acne.
   b. Hay fever.

N. *Expanding health insurance coverage*

1. *Expanding public coverage*
   a. Expansions of Medicaid/SCHIP at the state level.
   b. National health insurance program: "Medicare for All."

2. *Expanding private group coverage through current employer-sponsored system*
   a. Financial incentives for employers to provide coverage.
   b. Employer mandates.
   c. New group insurance options, especially for small employers.

3. *Subsidizing purchase of private health insurance through tax credits and deductions*
   a. Individual tax credits/deductions to subsidize insurance premiums.
   b. Increased utilization of health savings accounts for certain types of health insurance.

O. *Racial/ethnic disparities in health*[25–27]

1. *Health equity* refers to providing care that does not vary in quality because of personal characteristics such as gender, age, ethnicity/race, geographic location, and socioeconomic status.

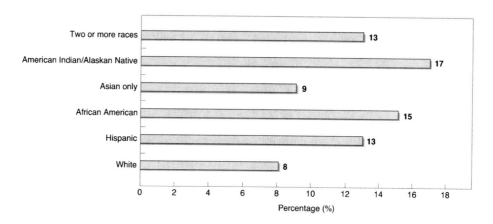

Figure 4-1   Percentage of Sample U.S. Residents with Fair or Poor Health by Race/Ethnicity, 2004

Race/Ethnicity	Nonpoor (%)	Near Poor (%)	Poor (%)
White (*n* = 166.6 million)	74	14	12
Hispanic (*n* = 40.8 million)	42	29	29
African American (non-Hispanic) (*n* = 32.6 million)	46	21	33
Asians only (*n* = 11.8 million)	68	16	17
American Indian/Alaska Native (*n* = 1.5 million)	43	23	34
Two or more races (*n* = 4.2 million)	59	20	21

Table 4-2   Poverty Status* of U.S. Residents, Age 65 and Younger, 2005

*The poverty status is based on the federal level (2005) of $19,971 for a family of four.

Source: Urban Institute and Kaiser Commission on Medicaid and the Uninsured, analysis of March 2006 Current Population Survey.

2. *U.S. population by race/ethnicity:* Whites make up the majority (67%), followed by Hispanics (14%), African Americans (non-Hispanic) (12%), Asian only (4%), two or more races (1%), American Indian/Alaskan Natives (0.7%), and Native Hawaiian/Pacific Islanders (0.1%).

3. African Americans and Hispanics, compared with Whites, are more likely to have uncontrolled diabetes and to present with short-term and long-term complications.

4. African Americans and Hispanics are more likely to be diagnosed with AIDS and to die from HIV infection, compared with Whites.

5. African Americans relative to Whites are less likely to experience increases in the quality of care.

VII. **Community Health Safety and Preparedness [PHCC.4.9]**

Public health, with its interdisciplinary approach to disease prevention and health promotions, plays a role in disaster preparedness by examining the impact of disaster on the population and by working with other agencies and organizations to incorporate the knowledge gained into planning for future responses.

A. *Core functions of public health*

1. Assessment and monitoring of the health of communities and populations at risk to identify health problems and priorities.

2. Formulating public policies, in collaboration with community and government leaders, designed to solve identified local and national health problems and priorities.

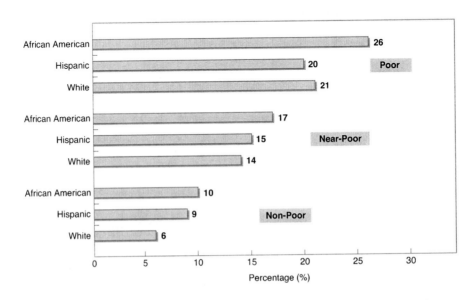

Figure 4-2   Sample of U.S. Residents with Fair or Poor Health by Race/Ethnicity and Poverty Status, 2004

3. Ensuring that all populations have access to appropriate and cost-effective care, including health promotion and disease prevention services, and evaluation of the effectiveness of that care.[27]

B. *Public Health Agencies' Obligations*[28]
    1. Prevent epidemics and the spread of disease.
    2. Protect against environmental hazards.
    3. Prevent injuries.
    4. Promote and encourage healthy behaviors and mental health.
    5. Respond to disasters and assist communities in recovery.
    6. Ensure the quality and accessibility of health services.

C. *Public health system:* a complex network of people, systems, and organizations.

D. *Goals*
    1. Improve health within the population.
    2. Strive to enhance the effectiveness with which health knowledge and technologies are applied to address the health issues of individuals and populations.
    3. Value equity in health and strive to reduce disparities in health across different social, economic, ethnic, and cultural groups.

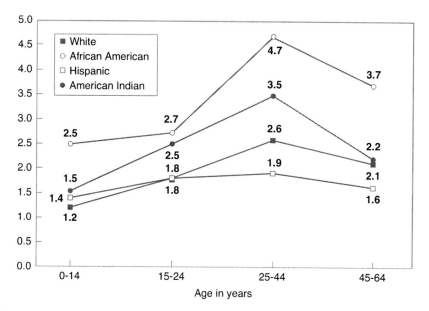

Figure 4-3 Mortality Ratio by Age and Race/Ethnicity, 2003

E. *Public health role in disasters*
1. Engage in planning for community protection and response.
2. Respond to disasters and assist communities in mitigation and recovery by:
   a. Ensuring that essential public health services are available and accessible.
   b. Rebuilding services that have been lost.
   c. Engaging community in plans for service delivery.
F. Ensuring the quality and accessibility of healthcare services involves:
1. Developing contingency plans for providing essential public health services.
2. Developing methods to ensure access to care and health services.
3. Ensuring access to care for non-disaster-related conditions.

VIII. **Organizational Problem Resolution: Organization and Management Theories [PHCC.4.10]**
A. *Systems thinking and systems tools*[29]
1. Concerns with understanding and guiding change in organizations, implying the examination of the overall structures, patterns, and cycles in systems, rather than focusing on isolated or specific events in the systems.
2. Understanding how systems thinking and tools are used in organization requires an understanding of a system in the first place.
   a. A system is an organized collection of parts that are highly integrated to accomplish an overall goal.
   b. The system has various inputs, which go through certain processes to produce certain outputs, which together accomplish the overall desired goal for the system.
3. Public health systems thinking reflects the potential of public health administrators/managers to identify solutions that address multiple problems within the system, hence maximizing improvement throughout the entire public health system (project or program).
4. Systems thinking implies long-term effects or solutions of an intervention and not short-term effects of public health intervention.

5. Further utilizing a bigger picture in the intervention model of public health initiative to control disease and promote health is also important.

   a. *Vignette:* Insect *A* causes cellulitis and insect *A* feeds on insect *B* (a potent pathogen for acute bacterial meningitis). Is systems thinking applied here by developing pesticides to eliminate insect *A* only?

   b. *Solution:* The approach to eliminating insect *A* only by developing a potent pesticide is not a systems thinking tool because the elimination of insect *A* will lead to a greater health problem—acute bacterial meningitis. Systems thinking will require integrated pest management, thus eliminating all insects associated with human health.

6. Systems thinking claims that:

   a. Parts of system communicate with each other.

   b. The system has an environment with communication entities.

   c. Systems are continuously changing, with a small stimulus causing a large effect or no effect at all (e.g., global warming).

   d. Systems behavior cannot be predicted from the behavior of its parts.

   e. A system as a whole works differently from its parts.

   f. Parts per se cannot accomplish what the system is capable of accomplishing; parts cannot contain the whole.

7. An organization is defined by complexity, and the systems that create that complexity are adaptive, implying organizational change and unpredictability of the future.

8. Public health problems are complex because there are so many factors that determine the health of the population. In effect, public health issues cannot be subjected to a simple cause-and-effect model.

9. Systems thinking claims to identify the real problems by going beyond the cause-and-effect model, thus providing potential solutions.

B. *Chaos theory*
1. Chaos theory deals with unpredictable complex systems.
   a. This theory originates, in part, from the work of Edward Lorenz, a meteorologist, who simulated weather patterns on a computer.
2. Rather than understanding a changing system as series of causal steps, chaos theory postulates a point in the system in the future, an attractor, which pulls the system so to speak toward it.
   a. When the system is unpredictable at a certain stage, the future may unfold quite differently, depending on what little difference occurred.
3. In public health organization and management, the chaos theory reflects the complexity and unpredictability of public health services because of its relations with other systems (state, federal government, local government, private sectors, etc.).

C. *Contingency leadership theory (CLT)*
1. CLT was proposed by the Austrian psychologist Fred Fiedler.
2. It classifies leaders into:
   a. Those motivated by the need to accomplish assigned tasks, implying task-oriented.
   b. Those motivated by close and supportive relations with members of the group (i.e., people-oriented).
3. The effectiveness of the leader is contingent upon:
   a. Leader's personality.
   b. Characteristics of the leadership situation.

D. Douglas McGregor's X-Y Theory
1. Douglas McGregor, an American social psychologist, proposed his famous X-Y theory in the 1960s.
2. McGregor's X-Y theory remains central to organizational development and to improving organizational culture.
3. McGregor's X-Y theory is indicative of the natural rules for managing people that, under the pressure of day-to-day business, are all too easily forgotten.
4. This theory maintained that there are two fundamental approaches to managing people:
   a. Many managers tend toward Theory X and generally get poor results.

    b. Enlightened managers use Theory Y, which produces better performance and results and allows people to grow and develop.

BOX 4-2 MANAGEMENT/LEADERSHIP THEORIES

- *McGregor's Theory Y* involves the management of employees by assuming that they are highly motivated. For example, staff are allowed to time-shift their work hours to accommodate their family schedules as long as they show productivity.
- *McGregor's Theory X* assumes that employees are not satisfied with their job environment, but are motivated exclusively by their salaries.
- *Contingent Theory* operates by adopting the management strategy aimed at meeting the needs of all personnel in the department.

    E. *Path-goal theory of leadership* (Robert House, 1971)
1. Developed to describe the way that leaders encourage and support their followers in achieving the goals they have been set by making the path that they should take clear and easy.
2. Maintains that leaders can affect the performance, motivation, and satisfaction of a group by:
   a. Offering rewards after achieving the performance goal.
   b. Clarifying paths toward these goals.
   c. Removing obstacles or barriers to performance.
3. This theory identifies four types of leadership styles:
   a. Directive.
   b. Supportive.
   c. Participative.
   d. Achievement-oriented.

IX. Strategic Planning and Marketing in Public Health [PHCC.4.9]

    A. Strategic planning (SP) refers to the overall direction of the business, including marketing and decision making about production and operations, finance, human resource management, and other business issues.
1. Public health services involve managed care and personal health services. Health clinics are required to apply marketing

strategies in retaining clients, which includes not only the provision of services but also the facilitation of access to care and services, including transportation for appropriate utilization of available services such as childhood immunization.

B. The objective of SP is to set the direction of a business and create its shape so that the products and services it provides meet the overall business objectives.

1. The essential public health services provide the outlines of public health services, which reflect the overall substance of public health, disease control and prevention, and health promotion. Public health services must be conducted with the overall goal of disease prevention and health promotion, thus fulfilling the mission of public health.

C. Marketing plays a major role in strategic planning, because it is the job of marketing management to understand and manage the links between the business and the "environment."

D. Public health practitioners work with the community in a marketing manner through outreach in order to provide services in the community and bring the community to the public health clinics. Public health can achieve its objectives through well-organized marketing planning.

E. This involves the effort of public health directors and managers in addressing the obvious questions relevant to SP and marketing strategies:

1. Where are we now? This provides data on the current/instant assessment of the project or services (e.g., a childhood immunization project).

2. How did we get there? This is addressed by comparing the baseline with the ongoing activities from the initiation of the project (e.g., the immunization rate of 80% of children eligible for a given vaccine).

3. Where are we heading? Direction, which must be reflected by the specific service objectives of the project such as childhood immunization (e.g., to increase the immunization rate by 10% by the year 2010).

4. Where would we like to be? This addresses the outcome of services from the baseline measure (e.g., to reduce the inci-

dence of childhood vaccine–preventable disease from 10% to 5% by the year 2010).

5. How do we get there? This is addressed by what services, resources, and manpower are needed to increase the immunization rate.

6. Are we on course? What are the data from the process evaluation of the immunization services?

F. In summary, SP and marketing planning applies to public health services through process, impact, and outcome evaluations, which must always be achieved if public health is to continue and maintain its place in the arena of disease prevention, control, and health promotion. And like business, public health services must operate by effectively maintaining surveillance and monitoring, obtaining the resources needed to invest in MCH, mobilizing the community, involving community leaders and stakeholders in decision making, establishing objectives and strategies to deliver services, and measuring performance (process and impact evaluation).

X. **Quality and Performance Improvement in Public Health Services [PHCC.4.4]**
   A. Based on the 10 essential public health services.
   B. Focus on overall public health system.
   C. Describe the optimal level of performance.
   D. Support a process of quality improvement.[30]
   E. *Essential public health services*[31]
      1. Monitor health status.
      2. Diagnose and investigate health problems.
      3. Inform, educate, and empower people.
      4. Mobilize communities to address health problems.
      5. Develop policies and plans.
      6. Enforce laws and regulations.
      7. Link people to needed health services.
      8. Ensure a competent workforce—public health and personal care.
      9. Evaluate health services.
      10. Conduct research for new innovations.
   F. System focus.

G. Because all entities contribute to the health and well-being of the community, public health must focus on system.

H. *Optimal level of performance*
1. Each performance standard represents the "gold standard."
2. Provide benchmarks to which state and local systems can strive to achieve.
3. Stimulate higher achievement.

I. *Quality improvement*
1. Standards should result in identification of areas for improvement.
2. Link results to an improvement process.[32,33]

XI. **Program Planning, Development, Conduct, and Evaluation [PHCC.4.8]**

A. Program development involves:
1. Planning.
2. Implementation.
3. Evaluation.

B. A logic model is efficient in examining program action:
1. *Input.*
2. *Outputs*
   a. Activities.
   b. Participation.
3. *Outcomes*
   a. Short-term impact.
   b. Medium-term impact.
   c. Long-term impact.

C. Program evaluation involves:
1. Data collection.
2. Analyses and interpretation.
3. Results.

D. *Example of program development: prostate cancer screening project*
1. Program input reflects the money, staff, research, and partners.
2. Program output reflects the educational materials for prostate risk reduction, sessions, and facilities to support the educational sessions.
3. The outcomes are knowledge gained, skills developed, and risk reduction as well as prostate cancer early diagnosis and mortality reduction.

E. The evaluation in logic model focuses on:
1. Assessment of needs and assets.
2. Process evaluation, which attempts to addresses the question: Are the sessions for prostate cancer education delivered as planned?
3. Outcome evaluation, which attempts to address the question: Is the prostate cancer screening program making a difference in terms of early diagnosis of prostate cancer?

F. *Reporting:* Program reporting in logic model provides data on:
1. Situation.
2. Response.
3. Results.
4. Evidence.

REFERENCES

1. United Kingdom Cabinet Office. *Professional Policy Making for the Twenty-First Century.* http://www.civilservant.org.uk/profpolicymaking.pdf. Accessed November 17, 2007.
2. Smith-Merry J, Gillespie J, Leeder SR. A pathway to a stronger research culture in health policy. *Aust New Zealand Health Policy.* 2007;4:19.
3. Hertzman C. Population health and human development. In: Keating D, Hertzman C, eds. *Developmental Health and the Wealth of Nations: Social, Biological and Educational Dynamics.* New York: Guilford Press; 1999:21–40.
4. Dahlgren G, Whitehead M. *Policies and Strategies to Promote Social Equity in Health.* Stockholm, Sweden: Institute for Future Studies; 1991.
5. Evans RG, Stoddart GL. Producing health, consuming healthcare. *Soc Sci Med.* 1990;31:1347–1363.
6. Berkman LF, Glass T. Social cohesion, social capital and health. In: Berkman LF, Kawachi I, eds. *Social Epidemiology.* New York: Oxford University Press; 2000:174–190.
7. McKinlay JB. The promotion of health through planned sociopolitical change: Challenges for research and policy. *Soc Sci Med.* 1993;36:109–117.
8. Kaplan GA, Everson SA, Lynch JW. The contribution of social and behavioral research to an understanding of the distribution of disease: a multilevel approach. In: Smedley BD, Syme SL, eds. *Promoting Health: Intervention Strategies from Social and Behavioral Research.* Washington, DC: National Academy Press; 2000:37–80.
9. Brownson RC, Newschaffer CJ, Ali-Abarghoul F. Policy research for disease prevention: challenges and practical recommendations. *Am J Public Health.* 1997; 87:735–739.

10. Geronimus AT. To mitigate, resist, or undo: addressing structural influences on the health of urban populations. *Am J Public Health*. 2000;90:867–872.

11. Milbank Memorial Fund, The National Association of State Budget Officers, and the Reforming States Group. *2002–2003 State Health Expenditure Report*, June 2005.

12. KFF/Harvard School of Public Health, *Health Care Agenda for the New Congress*, conducted November 4–28, 2004.

13. Kulynych J, Korn D. The new HIPAA (Health Insurance Portability and Accountability Act of 1996) Medical Privacy Rule: help or hindrance for clinical research? *Circulation*. 2003;108:912–914.

14. Kulynych J, Korn D. The effect of the New Federal Medical–Privacy Rule on Research. *N Engl J Med*. 2002;346:201–204.

15. Kilbridge P. The cost of HIPAA compliance. *N Engl J Med*. 2003;348:1423–1424.

16. Califf R, Muhlbaier L. Health Insurance Portability and Accountability Act (HIPAA): Must there be a trade-off between privacy and quality of health care or can we advance both? *Circulation*. 2003;108:915–918.

17. Department of Health and Human Services Rules and Regulations 45 CFR 46. *Federal Register* 46 (January 27, 1981); revised 1983, to include Subpart D: Research Involving Children; *Federal Register* 48 (March 4, 1983).

18. *Trials of War Criminals before the Nuremberg Military Tribunals under Control Council Law 10*. Washington DC: Superintendent of Documents, U.S. Government Printing Office; 1950.

19. World Medical Association. *Declaration of Helsinki*. 1964.

20. Sherav VH. Children in clinical research: A conflict of moral values. *Amer J Bioethics*. 2003;3(1):1–81. http://www.bioethics.net/journal/infocus/pdf/sharav.pdf. Accessed February 23, 2004.

21. Kaiser Permanente. *2003 Health Insurance Survey*. http://www.kff.org/insurance/loader.cfm?url=/commonspot/security/getfile.cfm&PageID=48503. Accessed November 21, 2007.

22. Fries JF, Koop CE, Sokolov J, Beadle CE, Wright D. Beyond health promotion: reducing need and demand for medical care. *Health Aff (Millwood)*. 1998;17: 70–84. doi: 10.1377/hlthaff.17.2.70.

23. Pollock AM, Rice DP. Monitoring health care in the United States—A challenging task. *Public Health Rep*. 1997;112:108–113.

24. Tengs TO, Adams ME, Pliskin JS, et al. Five-hundred life-saving interventions and their cost-effectiveness. *Risk Anal*. 1995;15:369–390. doi: 10.1111/j.1539-6924.1995.tb00330.x.

25. Murray CJ, Salomon JA, Mathers C. A critical examination of summary measures of population health. *Bull World Health Organ*. 2000;78:981–994.

26. Des J D.C., Jones A. Small world, big challenges: A report from the 9th International Congress of the World Federation of Public Health Associations. *Am J Public Health*. 2001;91:14–15.

27. Halfon N, Hochstein M. Life course health development: An integrated framework for developing health, policy, and research. *Milbank Q*. 2002;80:433–479.

28. U.S. Department of Health and Human Services. Office of Inspector General. *Work Plan Public Health Services Agencies Project.* http://oig.hhs.gov/reading/ workplan/1999/99phswp.pdf. Accessed October 15, 2007.

29. Free Management Library. *Systems Thinking.* http://www.managementhelp.org/ systems/systems.htm. Accessed February 14, 2008.

30. Centers for Disease Control and Prevention. http://www.cdc.gov/od/ocphp/ nphpsp/PresentationLinks.htm. Accessed April 30, 2008; http://www.phf.org/ performance.htm. Accessed April 30, 2008.

31. Institute of Medicine. *The Future of Public Health in the 21st Century.* Washington, DC: National Academy Press; 2003.

32. Centers for Disease Control and Prevention. http://www.cdc.gov/od/ocphp/ nphpsp/Documents/NPHPSP. Accessed March 28, 2008.

33. Centers for Disease Control and Prevention. http://www.cdc.gov/eval. Accessed April 29, 2008.

Chapter 5

Social and Behavioral Sciences in Public Health

Larry Holmes, Jr., and Doriel D. Ward

SOCIAL AND BEHAVIORAL SCIENCES CORE COMPETENCIES LEARNING OBJECTIVES

The social and behavioral sciences in public health address the behavioral, social, and cultural factors related to individual and population health and health disparities over the life course. Research and practice in this area contribute to the development, administration, and evaluation of programs and policies in public health and health services to promote and sustain healthy environments and healthy lives for individuals and populations.

PHCC.5.1.   Describe the role of social and community factors in both the onset and solution of public health problems.

PHCC.5.2.   Identify the causes of social and behavioral factors that affect the health of individuals and populations.

PHCC.5.3.   Identify basic theories, concepts, and models from a range of social and behavioral disciplines that are used in public health research and practice.

PHCC.5.4.   Apply ethical principles to public health program planning, implementation, and evaluation.

PHCC.5.5.   Specify multiple targets and levels of intervention for social and behavioral science programs and/or policies.

PHCC.5.6.   Identify individual, organizational, and community concerns, assets, resources, and deficits for social and behavioral science interventions.

PHCC.5.7.	Apply evidence-based approaches in the development and evaluation of social and behavioral science interventions.
PHCC.5.8.	Describe the merits of social and behavioral science interventions and policies.
PHCC.5.9.	Describe steps and procedures for the planning, implementation, and evaluation of public health programs, policies, and interventions.
PHCC.5.10.	Identify critical stakeholders for the planning, implementation, and evaluation of public health programs, policies, and interventions.

PREVIEW

Behavioral science, which embraces psychology, sociology, and anthropology, has been described as the study of actions and reactions of humans and other animals, using experimental and observational methodologies. The application of these disciplines to the health of the population represents its affiliation with public health. The behavioral and social sciences in public health address the behavioral, social, and cultural factors related to individual and population health and health disparities over the life cycle. Research and practice in this area contribute to the development, administration, and evaluation of programs and policies in public health and health services to promote and sustain healthy environments and healthy lives for individuals and populations. Therefore, behavioral science is a cross-fertilization between applied public health disciplines and management and policy sciences.

To maintain that there are rarely any health conditions without a behavioral input or influence is as true as maintaining that to every physical disease process, there is an emotional reaction. The role of behavior in risk and predisposing factors to acute and chronic diseases has been well illustrated, as well as the application of behavioral interventions in reducing disease risk factors, increasing compliance to intervention and treatment regimens, and improving disease prognosis and reducing mortality. Whereas the specific mechanisms have not been fully understood, it is plausible that behavior intervention, involving knowledge of health-related events risk or predisposing factors, may enhance skills toward risk avoidance or compliance to treatment, and hence improve the overall health outcomes. The social determinants of health have been clearly demonstrated. Inequity in education, income, and socioeconomic status (SES) has been associated with variances in disease presentation, screening, treatment received, and health outcome (including mortality). This chapter presents the basic concepts in behavioral sciences and their relations to health promotions, health theories and models (e.g., the theory of reasoned action), social and psychological determinants of health, and health disparities. Mention is made of ethical principles in program development, implementation, and evaluation. The factors influencing health at individual and population levels are highlighted. An evidence-based approach to public health program development and program evaluation is presented with the intent to emphasize the role of the community in the science-driven approach to health improvement.

I. **Behavioral Sciences and Its Role in Health Promotions and the Prevention of Health-Related Events [PHCC.5.1, 5.2]**
    A. *Health* and *disease* are determined by dynamic interactions among biological, psychological, behavioral, and social factors or variables.[1-3]
        1. These interactions occur over time and throughout the life cycle.
    B. The health of the public is integrally linked to social, behavioral, physical, biological, and economic environments.[4,5]
    C. *Psychological factors* influence health directly through biological mechanisms and indirectly through arrays of behaviors.

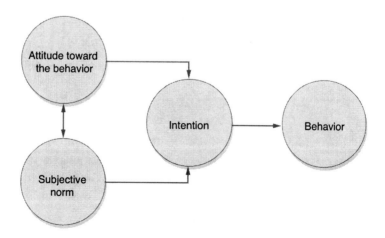

Figure 5-1 Theory of Reasoned Action

D. *Social and psychological factors* that influence health include: (1) SES, (2) social inequalities, (3) social network and support, (4) work conditions, (5) depression, (6) anger, and (7) hostility.[5,6]

E. *Behavior,* which is the collectivity of acts, is fundamental to health outcomes, health promotion, and disease prevention.

F. *The Healthy People 2010 initiative* demonstrates the potentials for change in behavior or behavior modification in reducing morbidity and mortality in most of the leading causes of death in the United States.[7]

G. *Behavioral sciences* refers to a multidisciplinary (sociology, anthropology, psychology) approach to the study of actions and reactions of humans and other animals through observational and experimental methods.

H. The behavioral sciences dimension of public health involves the use of sociologic, anthropologic, and psychological methodologies in understanding health behaviors and the application of this knowledge in designing interventions to promote health and prevent diseases, injuries, and disabilities (health-related events).

I. Whereas the substance of public health is disease prevention and health promotion, social sciences enhances health promotions by indicating:[8–10]

1. How people think about their behavior.
2. How people determine their risk (risk perception).
3. How people change their behavior.
4. How people cope with health issues/problems.

J. *Behavior change:* Deciding to change behavior depends on:

1. Beliefs about current health status
   a. General health values.
   b. Risk perception.
   c. Vulnerability.
   d. Self-efficacy.
   e. Response efficacy.
2. Impression management, which implies the influence of one's health behavior from the social perspective of one's behavior.
3. Intentions versus willingness, with willingness as a better predictor of behavior change relative to the intention to change behavior.

Table 5-1   The Importance of Behavior in Health , Morbidity, and Mortality, Healthy People 2010[7]

- The major leading causes of death (heart disease, cancer, and stroke) in the United States are associated with behavioral (lifestyle) variables.
- Reduction in heart disease morbidity and mortality can be achieved through smoking cessation, cholesterol lowering (dietary regulation), and exercise (physical activities).
- Significant decline in cancer death (lung, renal) can be achieved through smoking cessation.
- Substantial reduction in stroke can be achieved by controlling hypertension, regular exercise, dietary regulation, and smoking cessation.
- Significant reduction in auto accident mortality can be achieved by eliminating drunk driving.

K. *Health determinants* (illustrative): The key determinants of health include biological, social, behavioral, and psychosocial variables or factors, which may be illustrated as follows: [**PHCC.5.2**]

    1. *Hereditary:* Genetic predisposition plays an important role in obesity, most tumors, some chronic diseases, and emotional disorders such as schizophrenia. For example, prostate cancer tends to run in families, which is indicative of the possible role of gene, physical environment, or gene-environment interaction.[11,12]

    2. *Childhood development:* Chronic diseases such as childhood hypertension have been associated with early uterine and early developmental effects. For example, the failure to thrive has consequences beyond childhood.

    3. *Gender:* Gender predisposes to some behavioral risk factors and health conditions.[13,14] For example: (a) Men are more likely to be aggressive compared with women; studies using the Y chromosome explain this variation in aggressiveness. (b) Early-onset hypertension is more common in men than in women. (c) Autoimmune disorders such as systemic lupus erythematosus (SLE) are more common in women than men. Whereas no reliable explanation for the gender variation is available for SLE, it is plausible to suggest the role of estrogen, as well as

screening bias, because men are less likely to seek medical care and as such are less likely to be diagnosed relative to women.

4. *Coping skills:* Teaching individuals more adaptive coping skills may help reduce risky behavior.

5. *Personal health practices:* For example, breast self-examination may help discover breast lumps or cysts and may help in the diagnosis of early-stage breast tumors.

6. *Social environment:* Interpersonal relationships in family and social network settings have been shown to improve health conditions.

7. *Physical environment:* Environmental exposure influences the likelihood of developing a disease. For example,
   a. Cancers and asthma have been linked to air pollutants (tobacco and asbestos).
   b. Childhood neurologic deficit has been associated with exposure to lead-based paints.

8. *Employment status and working condition or environment:* Being unemployed is associated with impecunity, which influences access to health care, thus compromising screening and early diagnosis of treatable conditions (e.g., breast cancer, prostate cancer). Also, being employed and not having health insurance through that employment may increase the risk of morbidity for the same reason—reduced access to care. Further, uncomfortable working conditions may lead to a predisposition to stress in the first place and subsequent clinical conditions associated with high stress (hypertension, angina pectoris, coronary artery disease).[15–18]

9. *Educational status:* Higher educational status is associated with employment, high income level, access and utilization of health care (racial/ethnic majority), and knowledge of risk factors (all races/ethnicity)—all of which are variables/factors associated with improved health outcomes.

10. *Social support network:* Improved health outcomes.

11. *Family support system:* Improved health outcomes.

12. *Income and social class status:* The most important determinant of health and disease prognosis and mortality is income, which translates to social class (higher, middle, and lower) not race/ethnicity.[13]

13. *Cultural and racial/ethnic background:* Membership in a racial/ethnic group is associated with incidence, prevalence, and disease prognosis, as well as mortality. Race/ethnicity is a complex phenomenon and, like education, is associated with income, employability, access, and utilization of health care and knowledge of risk factors. African Americans, relative to Caucasians, bear the burden of disease disproportionately because this group is less educated and is therefore less likely to be employed; 80% live below poverty level, lack health insurance coverage, are less likely to receive early diagnosis, and hence have poor prognosis and increased mortality from most causes of death relative to their Caucasian counterparts.[8,9,18,19]

14. *Age:* Chronologic (physical) age is associated with disease incidence, prevalence, and mortality. For example: (a) Children and elderly are more predisposed to infectious diseases because of the compromization of the immune system. (b) Elderly are more vulnerable to chronic disabilities and chronic diseases. (c) Children are vulnerable to leukemia (nonsolid tumors), whereas advancing age is associated with most tumors (except germ cell testicular neoplasm, with the peak age of onset at age 29 to 34 years).

15. *Access to health services:* Early diagnosis and improved prognosis.

16. *Utilization and quality of health care:* Early diagnosis and improved prognosis.

L. Health promotion is the combination of educational, organizational, policy, financial, and environmental supports to reduce disease, disability, and injury risk factors and to promote healthy lifestyles.

M. Health promotion is achieved by: [PHCC.5.5]
   1. Following an objective such as *Healthy People 2010.*
   2. Identifying healthy people who are engaged in risky behaviors.
   3. Assisting individuals in their pursuit of specific behavior change.
   4. Motivating people to change their actions and reactions.
   5. Providing intervention that increases the likelihood of success.

N. Behavior change is influenced by (1) predisposing factors, which are: (a) knowledge, (b) beliefs, (c) attitudes, (d) gender, (e) age, (f) race/ethnicity, and (g) SES; (2) enabling factors, including

(a) skills and abilities and (b) available resources; and (3) reinforcing factors, such as (a) family support system, (b) social support network, and (c) motivation, or wanting or willingness to change behavior.

O. Behavior change strategies: (1) shaping, (2) visualization, (3) modeling, (4) controlling the situation, (5) reinforcement, (6) self-talk changing (improving one's image to encourage the change in behavior), (7) self-assessment, (8) personal behavior analysis, (9) decision making, and (10) realistic goal setting.

II. **Health Demographics and Health Disparities (Inequity)**[20,21]

A. *U.S. Demographics:* The U.S. population by race and Hispanic origins, for 2000 and projected for 2050, indicates that:

1. In 2000, non-Hispanic Whites totaled 274,595,678, more than two-thirds (75.1%) of the total population ($n = 281,421,906$).

2. By the year 2050, the U.S. Census Bureau predicts the proportion of the population that is non-Hispanic White will diminish to just more than half the total population.

3. Black or African Americans totaled 34,658,190, less than one-fifth (12.3%) of the total population.

4. American Indians/Alaska Natives (AI/AN) totaled 2,475,956 (0.9%) of the total population.

5. African American and AI/AN populations are also expected to increase.

6. Asian Americans totaled 10,242,998, and Native Hawaiian/Pacific Islanders (AAPI) totaled 398,835 (3.6% and 0.1%, respectively) of the total population.

7. The largest increase is expected in the AAPI population, which is expected to almost triple its current size by 2050.

8. Hispanics or Latinos totaled 35,305,818, and non-Hispanics or Latinos totaled 246,116,088 (12.5% and 87.5%, respectively) of the total population.

9. The Hispanic/Latino population is expected to almost double by 2050.

B. *Racial disparities in health and the measure of disparities*[21]

1. *Health disparities* refers to absolute and relative differences, disease rates, and health outcomes affecting the health status of certain race/ethnic, age, and gender groups, as well as socioeconomic/social class and geographic area/locale (e.g.,

Blacks and American Indians have diabetes at higher rates than Whites).

2. *Absolute and relative inequalities* (racial/socioeconomic model)
    a. The health gap between racial/socioeconomic groups can be considered in both relative and absolute terms.
    b. *Relative measure:* An example of a relative measure would be the ratio of the death rate in the lowest social class or one racial group (White) to that in the highest class/other racial groups (Black, Asian, Hispanic, or Latino).
    c. Death rates could be, for example, twice as high in Blacks as in Whites.

3. *Absolute measure* refers to the rate difference, which is computed by subtracting the death rate in one group from that in another (rate difference).
    a. This could be expressed as, for example, the death rate in Blacks (rates in Blacks = 75 deaths per 100,000) is 50 deaths per 100,000 greater than the rate in Whites (rates in Whites = 25 deaths per 100,000).
    b. Both relative and absolute measures have important implications.
    c. Absolute measures are the most critical (program planning and intervention), particularly with respect to identifying the major problems that need to be addressed. This is because an absolute measure is determined not only by how much more common the health problem is in one group than another, but also by how common the underlying problem (e.g., the death rate in a particular population) actually is.

C. *Racial and ethnic minority populations* [PHCC.5.2][22]
    1. Dramatic and persistent health disparities have been described among the following groups:
        a. *AI/AN:* people having origins in any of the original peoples of North and South America (including Central America), and who maintain tribal affiliation or community attachment.
        b. *Asian American:* people having origins in any of the original peoples of the Far East, Southeast Asia, or the Indian subcontinent.

   c. *Black or African American:* people having origins in any of the black racial groups of Africa.

   d. *Hispanic or Latino:* people of Cuban, Mexican, Puerto Rican, South or Central American, or other Spanish culture or origin, regardless of race.

   e. *Native Hawaiian or Other Pacific Islander:* people having origins in any of the original peoples of Hawaii, Guam, Samoa, or other Pacific Islands.

2. Disparities in health are observed in racial/ethnic background, with discrimination and bias of healthcare providers indicated as playing a fundamental role, illustrated as follows:

   a. Blacks are less likely than Whites to receive certain procedures and treatment (after controlling for income, education, and personal characteristics).

   b. Clinicians (doctors) in a study rated Blacks as less intelligent, less educated, more likely to use drugs and alcohol, less apt to comply with medical advice, and more likely to lack social support.

   c. Among Medicare recipients in managed care health plans, Blacks were less likely to receive (1) breast cancer screening, (2) eye exams when diabetic, (3) medicine after heart attack, (4) flu shots, and (e) follow-up care after hospitalization for mental illness.

   d. Asthmatic African Americans in one health maintenance organization were less likely than Whites to see specialists and to use inhalers and were more likely to be hospitalized.

   e. Blacks with diabetes are less likely to get proper medical care than White diabetics.

D. *Racial disparities in major causes of death and other conditions for disparities elimination*

1. *Age-adjusted mortality rates* (U.S., 2002) per 100,000 persons by race/ethnicity for three health focus areas (heart disease, cancer, stroke):

   a. African Americans have the highest all-cause death rate (1,083.3 per 100,000) and the highest death rate for three of the leading causes of death. They also lead in deaths from diabetes (49.5 vs. 25.4 per 100,000 for all populations); homicide (21.0 vs. 6.1 per 100,000 for all populations); influenza and pneumonia (24.0 vs. 22.6 per 100,000 for all populations); and breast, prostate, and lung cancer (34.0, 62.0, and 61.9 vs. 25.6, 27.9, and 54.9, respectively, per 100,000 for all populations).

b. African Americans have a higher cancer death rate than White Americans, even though White Americans have a higher prevalence of cancer: 7.8% for Whites, compared with 3.4% for African Americans, which is suggestive of some racial disparity in cancer screening and/or treatment.

c. African-American, American Indian, and Puerto Rican infants have higher death rates than White infants. In 2000, the Black-to-White ratio in infant mortality was 2.5 (up from 2.4 in 1998). This widening disparity between Black and White infants is a trend that has persisted over the past two decades.

d. African-American women are more than twice as likely to die of cervical cancer as are White women and are more likely to die of breast cancer than are women of any other racial or ethnic group.

e. Heart disease and stroke are the leading causes of death for all racial and ethnic groups in the United States. In 2000, rates of death from diseases of the heart were 29% higher among African-American adults than among White adults, and death rates from stroke were 40% higher.

f. In 2000, American Indians and Alaska Natives were 2.6 times more likely to have diagnosed diabetes compared with non-Hispanic Whites, African Americans were 2.0 times more likely, and Hispanics were 1.9 times more likely.

g. Although African Americans and Hispanics represented only 26% of the U.S. population in 2001, they accounted for 66% of adult AIDS cases and 82% of pediatric AIDS cases reported in the first half of that year.

h. In 2001, Hispanics and African Americans aged 65 and older were less likely than non-Hispanic Whites to report having received influenza and pneumococcal vaccines.

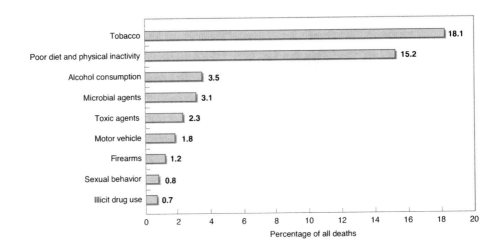

Figure 5-2   Leading Predisposing Factors of Death (Actual Causes) in the United States, 2002

Source: Mokdad AH, Marks JS, Stroup DF, Gerberding JL. Actual causes of death in the United States, 2000. *JAMA.* 2004;291:1238–1245.

E.   *Other health disparities measures* **[PHCC.5.2, 5.3]**

1.   Health disparities have been described among other populations, namely:

a.   SES.

b.   Geography (urban or rural).

c.   Gender.

d.   Age.

e.   Disability status.

f.   High-risk status related to sex and gender.

F.   *Sources of disparities in health*

1. Ethnicity and race (income, poverty).

2. Racial/ethnic discrimination (clinician's bias and prejudice).

3. Lack of and limited insurance coverage (income).

4. Lack of access to transportation and other barriers to access to health services (income).

5. Health services utilization (income).

6. Access and utilization of quality care (income).

7. Lifestyle variables.

8. Cultural variations.

9. Dietary patterns (income and lifestyle).

10. Lack of exercise.

11. Obesity and overweight.
12. Inadequate maternal and child health (poverty).
13. Environmental factors (income, which determines where individuals reside).
14. Stress and mental health (income and utilization of preventive health services).

G. *Barriers to eliminating racial disparities in health*
  1. Tuskegee experiment.
  2. Segregation of medical facilities and healthcare providers.
      a. These barriers result in distrust and reluctance to seek care.

H. *Eliminating disparities*
  1. Enforcing Title VI of the Civil Rights Act of 1964, which applies to healthcare providers who receive federal funds or other assistance from the U.S. Department of Health and Human Services (DHHS).[23]
  2. Title VI protects persons of every race (Black, White, Asian), color (skin color regardless of race), and national origin from unlawful discrimination.
  3. *Statement of Title VI:* Recipients of federal financial assistance (hospitals, nursing homes, home health agencies, managed

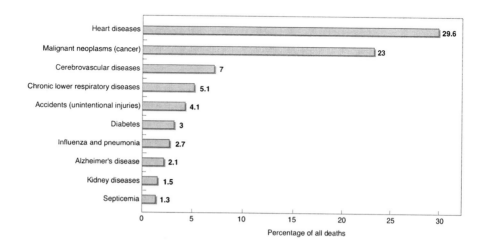

Figure 5-3 Leading Causes of Death in the United States, 2002

Source: National Center for Health Statistics. *Mortality Report.* Hyattsville, MD: U.S. Department of Health and Human Services; 2002.

care organizations, health research organizations, physicians, dentists, hospital social workers, as well as other providers who receive federal financial assistance from DHHS) may not, on the basis of race, color, or national origin, deny an individual a service, aid, or other benefit; provide a benefit that is different or provided in a different manner; subject an individual to segregation or separate treatment; restrict an individual in the enjoyment of benefits or privileges; treat an individual differently in determining eligibility; and/or deny a person an opportunity to participate on a planning or advisory board.

4. The DHHS has selected six focus areas in which racial and ethnic minorities experience serious disparities in health access and outcomes: (a) infant mortality, (b) cancer screening and management, (c) cardiovascular disease, (d) diabetes, (e) HIV/AIDS, and (f) immunizations.

5. Ethnic minorities are disproportionately affected by tuberculosis (TB), syphilis, mental illness, and hepatitis. For example, in 2002, 50% of those infected with Hepatitis B were AAPIs. Black teenagers and young adults become infected with Hepatitis B three to four times more often than those who are White.

6. Designing interventions to address these conditions is imperative for health disparities elimination.

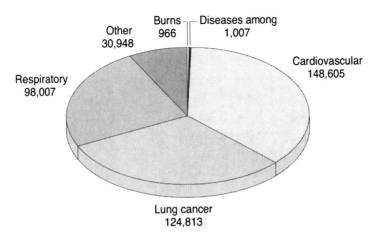

Figure 5-4 Major Diseases Caused by Smoking and Estimated Annual Number of Deaths, 1995–1999

Source: *Morbidity and Mortality Weekly Report (MMWR)*. 2002;51(14):300–303.

III. **Health Surveys and Behavior Interventions to Promote Health and Prevent Diseases [PHCC.5.5, 5.8]**
   A. Health surveys serve to gather information on health behaviors, including factors that influence, measure, or are affected by an individual's health.
   B. Health surveys are essential for the understanding of how psychological, behavioral, and social factors interact to define health risk behaviors and health.
   C. Health surveys serve as an important source of information for public health professionals; healthcare policymakers; private healthcare providers; and healthcare consumers concerned with planning, implementing, and evaluating health-related programs and policies.
   D. Health surveys may be classified according to: (1) characteristics of environment (political, cultural, social, economic, and physical), (2) population characteristics (demographics, resources, attitudes, knowledge, behavior—acts and reactions), (3) healthcare system characteristics (organizations, programs, insurers, professionals), (4) health status (physical, mental, social), (5) services utilization (type, site, purpose, time interval), (6) expenditures (total, out-of-pocket), and (7) satisfaction status (overall, general, visit-specific).
   E. Examples of health surveys that serve as sources of health data include:
      1. *National Health Interview Survey (NHIS):* conducted by the National Center for Health Statistics (NCHS).
         a. The NHIS is the leading source of health information on the civilian, noninstitutionalized population in the United States.
         b. The NHIS has been conducted annually since 1957 by the NCHS of the Centers for Disease Control and Prevention (CDC).
         c. In-person interviews of the NHIS core questionnaire are used to collect data on demographic, socioeconomic, and healthcare service access characteristics as well as health-related information on everyone in the household.
      2. *Behavioral Risk Factor Surveillance System (BRFSS):* provides state-specific information about issues such as asthma, diabetes,

healthcare access, alcohol use, hypertension, obesity, cancer screening, nutrition and physical activity, tobacco use, and more.

    a. The BRFSS is the world's largest ongoing telephone health survey system, tracking health conditions and risk behaviors in the United States yearly since 1984.

    b. It is conducted by the 50 state health departments as well as those in the District of Columbia, Puerto Rico, Guam, and the U.S. Virgin Islands, with support from the CDC.

3. *Health survey:* operational steps in design and conduct.

    a. Conceptualization of the topic for survey.

    b. Relating survey design to the objectives of the survey.

    c. Variable ascertainment.

    d. Reflection on the relationship between variables.

    e. Selecting data collection method.

    f. Sampling procedure.

    g. Research question formulation.

    h. Questionnaire formulation.

    i. Survey conduct or performance including monitoring and data safety.

    j. Data cleaning and editing.

    k. Analysis planning and performance (prescreening analysis and hypothesis-specific analysis).

    l. Results interpretation.

    m. Report preparation.

4. Behavioral intervention research involves the notion that behavior can be changed.

    a. Interventions to address risky behaviors such as smoking cessation, poor dietary patterns, and physical inactivity have been shown to be efficacious.

    b. These studies have utilized standard methodology that determines efficacy of intervention studies. The translation of these interventions from efficacy in the trial to effectiveness in the community settings involves the understanding of the following:

        (1) Which location or agent would work best in the implementation?

        (2) How many people would choose to use a program that has not been fully evaluated?

5. The basis of behavioral intervention is the consistent indication of behavior change.

    a. Behavioral interventions can successfully teach new behavior:

       (1) Behavioral interventions can successfully attenuate risky behaviors.

       (2) Maintaining behavior over time, however, is a greater challenge.

       (3) Short-term changes in behavior are encouraging, but improved health outcomes will often require prolonged interventions and lengthy follow-up.

       (4) Intervention studies are needed to evaluate the efficacy and effectiveness of modifying health risk behaviors.

    b. Intervention studies should span the breadth of all phases of clinical trials, from feasibility studies to randomized double-blinded studies.

    c. Intervention should include all levels of participants, from individual to family, community, and society.

    d. Behavioral and psychosocial interventions should be long term for optimal outcome.

    e. Individual behavior, family interactions, community and workplace relationships and resources, and public policy all contribute to health and influence behavior change.

    f. Interventions at multiple levels (individual, family, community, society) are more likely to sustain behavioral change.

    g. Interventions should address psychosocial factors associated with health status, such as access to healthy food and safe places to exercise, as well as individual behavior.

    h. Changes are necessary for improvement and maintenance of population health: [PHCC.5.8]

       (1) Social factors.

       (2) Policies.

       (3) Norms.

6. Analysis consideration:[24,25]

    a. Research studies, which are based on sample, make inference about the truth in the overall population.

    b. Some of the commonly used designs in studying health-risk behaviors include cross-sectional, or group comparison, longitudinal, and experimental designs.

   c. Essential to longitudinal design is predictive criteria, implying the prediction of changes over time.

   d. Concerns about longitudinal design:

     (1) Variations in the health indicator may be affected by other external factors in the environment.

     (2) Changes in the questions in the successive waves of study could introduce errors in detecting true changes in these indicators over time.

     (3) Improvement in diagnostic and treatment modalities or techniques for a selected illness can lead to a higher survival rate, thus a higher prevalence of the disease, over time.

   e. Multiple regression procedures may be used when two or more interval-level measures serve as predictors of some normally distributed interval-level dependent variable.

   f. In this model, the regression coefficient for any particular independent or explanatory variable (X_1) represents the change in the response or dependent variable (Y) associated with a one-unit change in X_1, while controlling for or maintaining other predictors (X_2, X_3, etc.) at constant.

   g. *Assumptions:*

     (1) The dependent variable should be normally distributed around the prediction line.

     (2) All variables are interval, or ratio-scaled.

   h. A two-way analysis of variance:

     (1) An *F*-test statistic can be used to summarize the difference in the variances between the groups on the dependent variable (Y).

     (2) The greater the variance between the groups, compared with the variance within the groups, the more likely it is that the differences in X between the groups are statistically significant.

   i. The chi-square statistic is often used in behavioral data to test for relationships between variables. This procedure is based on the null hypothesis of no association or independence.

(1) Nonparametric procedure involving nominal data.

(2) Examines the difference between the distribution that is observed compared with the distribution that would be expected, assuming the variables are not related.

(3) The less the variance between the observed and expected, the less support there is for the null hypothesis that there is no relationship between the variable in the particular sample.

(4) The purpose of hypothesis testing is to permit generalizations from a sample to the population from which the sample came (source population). Therefore, hypothesis testing confirms or negates the assertion that the observed findings did not occur by chance alone but rather occurred because of a true or factual association between the outcome and independent variables.

(5) Whether parametric or nonparametric technique of analysis, two types of errors can occur from a study: (a) type I error or alpha error occurs when a significant association is found when indeed there is no association—false-positive error, implying the rejection of a *true-null* hypothesis; and (2) type II or beta error occurs when one wrongly concludes that there is no significant association, when indeed there is one—false-negative, implying the rejection of a *true-alternative* hypothesis.

(6) The *p* value or alpha level refers to the probability of type I error. Simply, *p* value is a measure of the strength of the evidence provided by the data in favor of the null hypothesis. By convention, the alpha level is set at 0.05 (5% error acceptance). Therefore, if the *p* value is < 0.05 (alpha level), then the evidence against the null hypothesis is strong enough for one to reject it and claim that the observed finding is significant.

(7) The *p* value limitations: (a) Gives no information about the strength/magnitude of association. (b) May be statistically significant but clinically irrelevant or unimportant.

(8) A 95% confidence interval provides information on the magnitude of the association as well as the precision, thus furnishing one with a range of values to interpret the implications of the result.

IV. **Health Theories and Health Beliefs [PHCC. 5.3, 5.8]**
   A. *Definitions*
      1. *Belief:* Refers to the appraisal of the relationship between some object, action, or idea and some attitude of that object, action, or idea. Beliefs may develop from direct or indirect experience.
      2. *Attitude:* Refers to a relatively stable set of beliefs, feelings, and behavioral tendencies in relation to someone or something.

BOX 5-1   HEALTH BELIEF MODEL VARIABLES

- The notion that health behaviors are motivated by health belief is fundamental to HBM.
- The variables or principles behind the application of this model are:
  - **Perceived Susceptibility**—history of testicular cancer in the family
  - **Perceived Severity**—higher mortality from testicular cancer may predispose to testicular cancer self examination (TCSE)
  - **Perceived Benefits**—if TCSE decreases incidence and leads to early stage diagnosis, then this benefit may increase TCSE
  - **Perceived Emotional barriers**—if the level of anxiety is low, then subjects may be more likely to practice TCSE
  - **Perceived Skills barriers**—if skills are developed or perceived to be there, this will enhance TCSE
  - **Self Efficacy**—having confidence in practicing TCSE will enhance further use of TSCE in monitoring testicular health

---

   B. *Health theories and models:* The theories and models used to account for this change include:
      1. *Health belief model*[26,27] (developed in 1966 by Rosenstock, a psychologist)
         a. This model maintains that when beliefs affect behavior change, several factors must support a belief before change occurs:
            (1) Perceived seriousness of the health problem.

(2) Perceived susceptibility to the health problem.

(3) Cues to action, which implies the influence of direct and indirect cues in making change.

2. *Theory of reasoned action (TRA)*

 a. Proposed by Fishbein[28] and Ajzen[29] in an attempt to establish a relationship among beliefs, attitudes, intentions, and behaviors.

 b. TRA is based on two assumptions: (1) humans are rational animals who possess the ability to process and use the information available for them, and (2) humans use the information they process to achieve a reasonable behavioral decision.

 c. According to TRA, the determinant of a person's behavior is his intention to either perform or not to perform the specific behavior.

  (1) Due to the difficulties of always determining a person's intention, the theory of reasoned action specified two conceptually independent factors that, interacting together and weighted for the relative importance of each, determine intention.[29,30]

  (2) The attitude toward the behavior means a personal factor that considers the degree to which a person has positive or negative attitudes about evaluating a specific behavior.

 d. Simply, behaviors result from our intention to perform actions.

 e. The subjective norm is a social factor that refers to the apprehended social pressure to either perform or not to perform the behavior in question.

 f. Simply, persons are influenced by the approval or disapproval of close friends, loved ones, and social groups.

3. *Theory of planned behavior*

 a. Adds to the theory of reasoned action the concept of perceived control over the opportunities, resources, and skills necessary to perform a behavior.

 b. The concept of perceived behavioral control is similar to the concept of self-efficacy, implying an individual's perception of his or her ability to perform the behavior.

       c.   Perceived behavioral control over opportunities, resources, and skills necessary to perform a behavior is believed to be a critical aspect of behavior change processes.

4.   *Transtheoretical model (TTM) of health behavior change*

       a.   Serves as the basis for developing effective interventions to promote health behavior change.

       b.   Proposed by Prochaska and DiClemente[31]; Prochaska, DiClemente, and Norcross,[32] and Prochaska and Velicer.[33]

       c.   TTM is an integrative model of behavior change that describes how people modify a problem behavior or acquire a positive behavior.

       d.   The central organizing construct of the model is the stages of change and includes a series of independent variables: the processes of change and a series of outcome measures, including the decisional balance and the temptation scales.

       e.   Interventions based on the TTM potentially have both a high efficacy and a high recruitment rate, thus dramatically increasing the potential impact on entire populations of individuals with behavioral health risks.

       f.   The stages of change as proposed in the model are as follows:

          (1) Pre-contemplation is the stage in which people are not intending to take action in the foreseeable future, usually measured as the next 6 months.

          (2) Contemplation is the stage in which people are intending to change in the next 6 months.

          (3) Preparation is the stage in which people are intending to take action in the immediate future, usually measured as the next month.

          (4) Action is the stage in which people have made specific overt modifications in their lifestyles within the past 6 months.

          (5) Maintenance is the stage in which people are working to prevent relapse but do not apply change processes as frequently as do people in action.

5.   *Social learning theory (social cognitive theory)*

       a.   Proposes that behavior change is affected by environmental influences, personal factors, and attributes of the behavior itself.

    b. Each may affect or be affected by either of the other two, with the central tenet of social cognitive theory being the concept of self-efficacy.

    c. A person must believe in his or her capability to perform the behavior (i.e., the person must possess self-efficacy) and must perceive an incentive to do so (i.e., the person's positive expectations from performing the behavior must outweigh the negative expectations).

    d. A person must value the outcomes or consequences that he or she believes will occur as a result of performing a specific behavior or action.

    e. Outcomes may be classified as having immediate benefits (e.g., feeling energized following physical activity) or long-term benefits (e.g., experiencing improvements in cardiovascular health as a result of physical activity).

       (1) Because these expected outcomes are filtered through a person's expectations or perceptions of being able to perform the behavior in the first place, self-efficacy is believed to be the single most important characteristic that determines a person's behavior change.

       (2) Self-efficacy can be increased in several ways, among them are providing clear instructions, providing the opportunity for skill development or training, and modeling the desired behavior.[34]

6. *Ecological theory of behavior change*

    a. Most theories and models of behavior change tend to emphasize individual behavior change process and pay little attention to sociocultural and physical environmental influences on behavior.

    b. Ecological approaches to increasing participation in an intervention focus on sociocultural and environmental influences on behavior.

    c. These approaches emphasize the creation of supportive environments as well as the development of personal skills and the reorientation of health services.

    d. An underlying theme of ecological perspectives is that the most effective interventions occur on multiple levels.

    e. A model has been proposed that encompasses several levels of influences on health behaviors: intrapersonal factors, interpersonal and group factors, institutional factors, community factors, and public policy.

f. Similarly, another model has three levels (individual, organizational, and governmental) in four settings (schools, worksites, healthcare institutions, and communities).

g. Interventions that simultaneously influence these multiple levels and multiple settings may be expected to lead to greater and longer-lasting changes and maintenance of existing health-promoting habits.

h. This is a promising area for the design of future intervention research to promote physical activity.

7. *Relapse prevention model*

a. Focuses on factors that contribute to relapse, including negative emotional or physiologic states, limited coping skills, social pressure, interpersonal conflict, limited social support, low motivation, high-risk situations, and stress.

b. Principles include identifying high-risk situations for relapse (e.g., change in season) and developing appropriate solutions (e.g., finding a place to walk inside during the winter).

Table 5-2   Similarities and Differences of the Behavior Change Theories and Models

Theory/Model	Description
Health belief	Highlights the role of the perceived outcomes of behavior, although different terms are used for this construct, including perceived benefits and barriers.
Social cognitive/ planned behavior	Highlights the role of the perceived outcomes of behavior, although different terms are used for this construct, including perceived benefits and barriers and outcome expectations.
Reasoned action and planned behavior	Emphasizes the influence of perceptions of control over behavior; this influence is given labels such as self-efficacy (health belief model, social cognitive theory) and perceived behavioral control.
Ecologic model	Emphasizes social support, interpersonal and environmental influences.

C. Some similarities can be noted among the behavioral and social science theories and models used to understand and enhance health behaviors such as physical activity.

D. Most of the theories and models, however, do not address the influence of the environment on health behavior.

V. **Behavioral Risk Factors in Major Diseases [Chronic Diseases; Cancer; Maternal and Child Health; Infant Mortality; Infectious Diseases, Including Sexually Transmitted Infections (STIs) and HIV; and Conditions (Obesity, Pregnancy)]**

A. *Predisposing, enabling, and reinforcing factors*

1. *Predisposing factors* in disease, disability, and injury include: (a) knowledge, (b) beliefs, (c) values, (d) attitudes, (e) culture, (f) socio-demographics (gender, age, income, education, marital status), and (g) access and utilization of the healthcare system.

2. *Enabling factors* in health include (a) skills and capabilities; (b) adequate support and resources; (c) health resources availability; (d) community and governmental support, prioritization, and commitment to health; (e) health-related skills; (f) physical, mental, and emotional capabilities; (g) time and financial resources; and (h) safe areas (environment).

3. *Reinforcing factors* in health include: (a) family support system; (b) social support network; (c) peer support; (d) employer actions and policies; (e) health provider cost and access, as well as low cost and utilization of quality health care; (f) access to public health and patient education; and (g) community resources.

4. Outcomes of interaction among predisposing, enabling, and reinforcing factors result in (a) regular health assessment, (b) weight management, (c) improved relationships (inter- and intrapersonal), (d) safer sexual behaviors, (e) safer drug use, (f) improved dietary patterns, (g) stress management and control, (h) improved consumer decisions, and (i) increased physical activities.

5. The outcome of the behavior change given a healthy interaction between predisposing, enabling, and reinforcing factors are reductions in (a) chronic disabilities, (b) STIs, (c) heart diseases, (d) cancer, (e) mortality due to auto accidents, and (f) infant and maternal mortality.

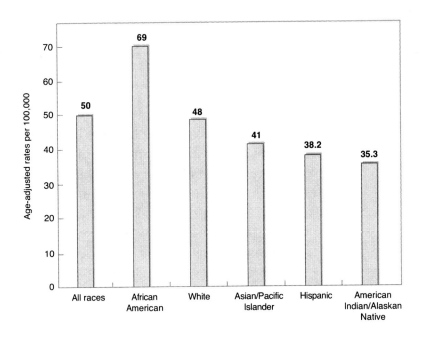

Figure 5-5 Age-Adjusted Mortality Rates per 100,000 Persons by Race/Ethnicity for Cerebrovascular Disease: United States, 2004

Source: Health US, 2006, www.cdc.gov/nchs/data/hus06.pdf#summary, Table 29.

B. Behavioral risk factors in major diseases and health indicators [PHCC.5.3]

1. Heart disease, malignant neoplasm, and stroke, which are chronic diseases, are the three leading causes of morbidity and mortality in the United States.

2. These conditions are linked with a limited number of health risk behaviors, such as cigarette smoking, poor nutrition, physical inactivity, and underuse of prevention practices.

3. Preventing and reducing the prevalence of health risk behaviors and subsequent morbidity and mortality attributed to chronic diseases remain major goals of public health.

4. The *Healthy People 2010* (HP 2010) objectives aim to reduce the impact of high-risk behaviors and increase use of preventive services.

C. *Basic notions in health risk behaviors*

1. Risk or predisposing factors to disease and disabilities are both modifiable and nonmodifiable.

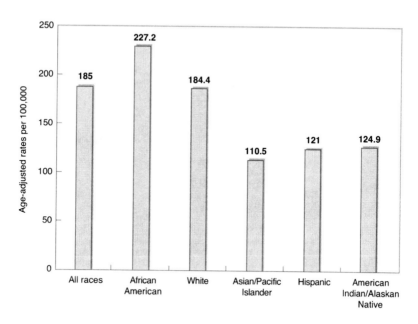

Figure 5-6   Age-Adjusted Mortality Rates per 100,000 Persons by Race/Ethnicity for Malignant Neoplasm: United States, 2004

Source: Health US, 2006, www.cdc.gov/nchs/data/hus06.pdf#summary, Table 29.

    2. Modifiable risk factors are those that are controllable or treatable, such as lifestyle and the lowering of serum cholesterol or glucose level by treatment compliance.

    3. Nonmodifiable risk factors are factors predisposing to disease that are uncontrollable such as age, gender, and race/ethnicity.

    4. Modifiable risk factors present a great potential for the control, reduction, and elimination of diseases.

    5. Behavior changes that affect lifestyle remain the hallmark of diseases that are associated with modifiable risks such as chronic diseases, chronic disabilities, and infectious diseases.

  D. Health risk behaviors (risk factors) associated with heart disease (first leading cause of mortality in the United States, representing 29.5% of the total causes of death in 2002); modifiable risk factors (health risk behaviors):[35,36]

    1. High blood cholesterol, mainly disproportional balance between high-density lipoprotein (HDL) and low-density lipoprotein (LDL), resulting in higher ratio of LDL to HDL.

    2. High blood pressure.

3. Smoking—accounts for nearly 30% of all deaths due to heart disease, as well as the leading predisposing factor to death in the United States (18.1%).
4. Physical inactivity.
5. Overweight and obesity.
6. Diabetes.

E. Health risk behaviors (risk factors) associated with stroke (third leading cause of death in the United States, representing 6.9% of the total cause of death in 2002); modifiable risk factors (health risk behaviors):
1. Smoking—active and passive.
2. Alcohol use.
3. Obesity.
4. Uncontrolled high blood pressure.
5. Physical inactivity.

F. Health risk behaviors (behavioral risk factors) associated with major malignant neoplasm (second leading cause of death in the United States, accounting for 22.9% of all deaths in 2002); modifiable risk factors (health risk behaviors):
1. Obesity and overweight (colon, endometrial, breast cancers).
2. Smoking—active and passive (renal, lung, oral cavity neoplasm).
3. Physical inactivity.
4. High-fat diet.
5. Alcohol consumption (oral cavity neoplasm).
6. Excessive exposure to ultraviolet radiation (sunlight).

G. *Diabetes mellitus:* Health risk behaviors include:
1. Physical inactivity leading to obesity.
2. Poor dietary habits.
3. Alcohol.
4. Smoking.
5. Obesity.

H. *Hypertension:* Health risk behaviors include:[36,37]
1. Physical inactivity.
2. High sodium intake.[37]
3. Impaired coping skills—stress management.
4. High-fat/lipid diet.
5. Lack of rest (inadequate sleep).
6. Excessive alcohol consumption.
7. Smoking.

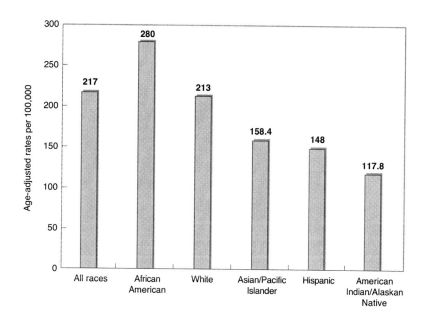

Figure 5-7   Age-Adjusted Mortality Rates per 100,000 Persons by Race/Ethnicity for Heart Disease: United States, 2004

Source: Health US, 2006, www.cdc.gov/nchs/data/hus06.pdf#summary, Table 29.

   I. *HIV/AIDS:* Health risk behaviors include:
      1. Drug and alcohol use.
      2. Unprotected sex.
      3. Multiple sexual partners.
      4. Lack of risk perception and self-efficacy.
      5. Exchange of sex for drugs or money.
   J. Inadequate health monitoring/screening and lack of health education are health risk behaviors that are associated with the preceding illustrative health conditions.

VI. Health Promotion Components and Levels of Disease Prevention
   A. Health promotion involves the following components:
      1. *Educational:* provision of information about risk behaviors and their consequences.
      2. *Organizational:* provision of programs and services that encourage participation and establish social support system.
      3. *Environmental:* provision of regulatory mechanisms to govern behavior and support behavior change or modification.
      4. *Financial:* provision of incentive such as monetary to maintain healthful behaviors.

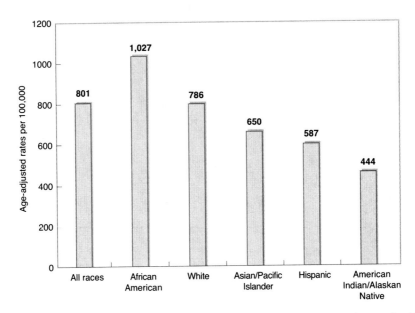

Figure 5-8   Age-Adjusted Mortality Rates per 100,000 Persons by Race/Ethnicity for All Causes of Death: United States, 2004

Source: Health US, 2006, www.cdc.gov/nchs/data/hus06.pdf#summary, Table 29.

B.   Disease prevention involves three basic levels:
   1.   *Primary prevention* refers to risk reduction and health problems avoidance in the first place.
   2.   *Secondary prevention* refers to the provision of intervention to reduce or eliminate risk or predisposing behaviors before the progression to clinical or overt disease state.
   3.   *Tertiary prevention* refers to the provision of treatment or rehabilitation after the event has already occurred in order to reduce its complications (e.g., stroke rehabilitation).

VII.   **Role of Social and Community Factors in Both the Onset and Solution of Public Health Problems [PHCC.5.1]**
   A.   Health is inextricably linked to an individual's status in society. This is the case regardless of the indicator used, be it income, education, or socioeconomic environment. An individual's relative economic and political power, or lack thereof, has been a determinant factor regarding access to resources supportive to health.
      1.   Community health promotion requires a comprehensive program, and community-based interventions may offer the most promising approach.[38]

B. When the social environment is the source of health problems, the solution to these problems lies in social change.
    1. Social change is best initiated by people and communities who have been empowered through education that raises consciousness of the social roots of their problems.[39]
C. The key to community mobilization for health promotion is the creation of viable partnerships between health educators and members and leaders of the community.
D. Self-efficacy theories offer many insights on how to develop more successful community mobilization programs.[40]

VIII. **Social and Behavioral Factors That Affect Health of Individuals and Populations [PHCC.5.2]**

Factors that affect primarily individuals include their personal attitudes toward disease determinants such as physical activity and dietary pattern; knowledge of disease risk factors, available services, and healthful behaviors; personal belief systems that affect disease screening, eating habits, and physical activity; self-perceived ability to make and sustain behavior changes; financial resources to access preventive health services, support healthy eating habits, and behavior changes; and reasons for desiring behavior change.

Factors that primarily affect population's or groups' health status include cultural beliefs that affect seeking a healthful behavior, availability of community resources to enhance lifestyle changes such as exercise facilities and equipment, financial resources necessary to provide healthier food, and physical activity choices.

A. Community and population factors create environments that can either promote or hinder behavior.
    1. Changes made by families or individuals.
    2. The presence or lack of safe places to be physically active as well as food venues that offer healthy food choices in reasonable portion sizes can either support or deter an individual's attempts to improve his or her health.
B. Policies regarding dietary patterns at schools and daycare centers influence eating habits as well as physical activities. For example, exposure to TV ads on food products shapes the individual's and community's notions of healthful diet.

C. *Personal factors influence health*
1. Knowledge, attitude, and beliefs.
2. Self-efficacy.
3. Motivation to cultivate a healthful lifestyle such as smoking cessation.
4. Psychosocial and motor skills development and potentials.
5. Cognitive potentials.

D. *Interpersonal factors*
1. Family and parental notion of health and behavior.

E. *Community and cultural factors*
1. Cultural norms and beliefs such as "what I don't know won't kill me," which hinders health screening in some segments of the U.S. population.
2. Availability of community centers for preventive health services and health education.

F. *Population influence*
1. Policy development in support of public health measures, advocacy, legislation, and industry regulation.
2. Environmental justice in the protection of health of the vulnerable populations from industries and governmental toxins (individuals in low SES groups tend to reside in environments with toxic waste).
3. The interaction of social structure and SES with other influences in complex pathways affects the health of individuals and communities, contributing to health disparities.
4. Social class, which reflects SES, has been indicated as an explanatory variable in racial health disparities, prenatal and early nutrition, and cognitive capacity.
5. Education, income, wealth, occupation, and other SES indicators are potent determinants of health.[41]

G. Determinants of health are multifactorial (web of causality) and reflect the complexities of disease process and factors driving these processes. In the early 1900s, deaths in the United States and Europe were primarily due to infectious diseases (mainly TB). The simplistic model of "one agent—one disease," implying a specific agent in disease causation, tends to explain the pathway of disease manifestation while dealing with pathogenic microbes. Surprisingly, the epidemiologic transition from infectious diseases to chronic diseases as a result of cardiovascular mortality due to cigarette smoking occurred before the onset of streptomycin in the treatment of TB in 1947.[42]

This experience is indicative of factors that may influence disease causation that are often ignored in the pathway. The reduction in TB mortality was achieved through public health effort made possible by increasing sanitation and adequate nutrition (potentiation of the immune system and hence inactivation of *mycobacterium tubaculae*), as well as through the decreased birth rate. Clearly, these factors influenced mortality by increasing the host immune responsiveness (thus inactivating the agent), limited the spread via sanitation, and restricted human contact (decrease in population growth). Public health efforts cannot be fully achieved without the inclusion of those who lack basic conditions necessary for good health, including safe housing, air, water, nutrition, working conditions, and access to medical care; these populations are ultimately the same people who organize to bring themselves better health conditions.[43] Risk factors in disease causation must consider the role that popular movements such as environmental justice can play in the improvement of public health.

IX. Ethical Principles to Public Health Program Planning, Implementation, and Evaluation [PHCC.5.4]

> *"Public health institutions should provide communities with the information they have that is needed for decisions on policies or programs and should obtain the community's consent for their implementation."*

> Public Health Leadership Society

A. Communities provide data for public health research, and the acquisition of such information must be achieved with informed consent from the onset of research, which involves: (a) community-based participatory research and (b) community advisory boards.

B. An approach to research in public health that portrays ethical consideration must evaluate at onset the outcome and the limitations such as sample size issues, blinding, and long-term follow-up, as well as the ethical issue of withholding results from the community.

C. Research design should begin with the development of the state-
    ment of the issue—a problem statement or research question—
    that is feasible.

D. Quantify the issue and indicate the method used to achieve the
    point estimate or some parameters (such as the prevalence of
    thoracolumbar kyphosis in children with achondroplasia).

E. Conduct a literature search (medline, pubmed, cancerlit,
    Cochrane database, etc.) on the issue and organize data.

F. Develop and prioritize program options.

G. Develop an action plan.

H. Mobilize the community and increase community participation.

I. Perform research, collect data, and manage data.

J. Conduct an analysis of clean data and communicate results to
    the community.

X. **Principles of Evidence-Based Public Health [PHCC.5.7] and Public
    Health Resources [PHCC.5.6]**

A. *Evidence-based public health (EBPH)* is the conscientious, explicit,
    and judicious use of current best evidence in making decisions
    about the care of communities and populations in the domain of
    health protection, disease prevention, health maintenance, and
    improvement.[44]

B. EBPH is the development, implementation, and evaluation of
    effective programs and policies in public health through applica-
    tion of principles of scientific reasoning, including systematic
    uses of data and information systems and appropriate use of pro-
    gram planning models.[45]

C. *Evidence-based medicine (EBM)* is the integration of best research
    evidence with clinical expertise and patient values.

D. This concept, which was developed in the early 1990s (before
    EBPH), came as the result of a large volume of literature and orig-
    inal articles on randomized clinical trials. The purpose was to
    apply the best available data in patient care.

E. EBM involves (1) converting the need for information into
    an answerable question, (2) tracking down the best evidence,
    (3) critically appraising that evidence, (4) integrating the
    appraisal with one's clinical expertise and the individual
    patient, and (5) evaluation.

    F. Epidemiology has been described as the foundation of both EBM and EBPH.[44]

    G. EBPH uses complex interventions with multiple community and societal issues in arriving at the best public health service.

    H. EBPH performance involves the following steps:

       1. Development of the problem narrative or initial statement of the issue.

       2. Search of the scientific literature.

       3. Organizing information to reflect the magnitude of the issue.

       4. Quantifying the issue (prevalence, incidence, relative risk, hazard ratio) using sources of existing data.

       5. Developing and prioritizing program options.

       6. Implementing interventions and projects.

       7. Evaluating the program or policy (process, impact, and outcome).[45]

    I. Public health encompasses the efforts, science, art, and approaches used by all sectors of society to ensure, maintain, protect, promote, and improve the health of the people.[46]

    J. Public health structure includes, but is not limited to, communities, the healthcare system, employers and businesses, the media, academia, and government.

       1. To meet the goals of public health, EBPH utilizes the following resources: (a) collaborative review groups, (b) methods groups, (c) fields, (d) consumer network, and (e) centers.

       2. Another important resource for EBPH is the Guide to Community Preventive Services (www.thecommunityguide.org). The Guide uses a defined, evidence-based approach to develop recommendations for addressing a number of important public health issues.

REFERENCES

1. Alonso A, Martinez-Gonzalez MA. Mediterranean diet, lifestyle factors, and mortality. *JAMA*. 2005;293:674–675.

2. Trichopoulou A, Costacou T, Bamia C, Trichopoulos D. Adherence to a Mediterranean diet and survival in a Greek population. *N Engl J Med*. 2003;348: 2599–2608.

3. Anderson CA, Appel LJ. Dietary modification and CVD prevention: a matter of fat. *JAMA*. 2006;295:693–695.

4. Berkman LF, Kawachi I. *Social Epidemiology.* New York: Oxford University Press; 2000.

5. Braveman PA, Cubbin C, Egerter S, et al. Socioeconomic status in health research: One size does not fit all. *JAMA.* 2005;294(22):2879–2888.

6. Feinstein JS. The relationship between socioeconomic status and health: A review of the literature. *Milbank Q.* 1993;71(2):279–322.

7. *Healthy People 2010: Understanding and Improving Health.* Washington, DC: U.S. Department of Health and Human Services; 2001.

8. House JS, Kessler RC, Herzog AR. Age, socioeconomic status, and health. *Milbank Q.* 1990;68(3):383–411.

9. Kitagawa EM, Hauser PM. *Differential Mortality in the United States: A Study of Socioeconomic Epidemiology.* Cambridge, MA: Harvard University Press; 1973.

10. Antonovsky A. Social class, life expectancy and overall mortality. *Milbank Mem Fund Q.* 1967;45(2):31–73.

11. Garcia-Closas M, Wacholder S, Caporaso N, Rothman N. Inference issues in cohort and case–control studies of genetic effects and gene–environment interactions. In: Khoury M, Little J, Burke W, eds. *Human Genome Epidemiology: A Scientific Foundation for Using Genetic Information to Improve Health and Prevent Disease.* Oxford, UK: Oxford University Press; 2004.

12. Greenland S, Rothman K. Concepts of interaction. In: Rothman K, Greenland S, eds. *Modern Epidemiology.* Philadelphia: Lippincott Williams & Wilkins; 1998.

13. Doyal L. *What Makes Women Sick? Gender and the Political Economy of Health.* London: Macmillan; 1995.

14. Clarke JN. Sexism, feminism and medicalism: A decade review of the literature on gender and illness. *Sociol Health & Illness.* 1983;5:62–82. doi: 10.1111/1467-9566.ep11340067.

15. Judge K, Mulligan J, Benzeval M. Income inequality and population health. *Soc Sci Med.* 1998;46:567–579.

16. Lynch J, Davey Smith G, Hillemeier M, Shaw M, Raghunathan T, Kaplan G. Income inequality, the psychosocial environment, and health: Comparisons of wealthy nations. *Lancet.* 2001;358:194–200.

17. Gravelle H, Wildman J, Sutton M. Income, income inequality and health: What can we learn from aggregate data? *Soc Sci Med.* 2002;54:577–589.

18. Ben-Shlomo Y, White I, Marmot M. Does the variation in the socioeconomic characteristics of an area affect mortality? *BMJ.* 1996;312:1013–1014.

19. Kaplan G, Pamuk E, Lynch J, Cohen R, Balfour J. Inequality in income and mortality in the United States: Analysis of mortality and potential pathways. *BMJ.* 1996;312:999–1003.

20. Senior PA, Bhopal R. Ethnicity as a variable in epidemiological research. *BMJ.* 1994;309:327–330.

21. Soto MA, Abel C, Diever A, eds. *Healthy Communities: New Partnership for the Future of Public Health.* Washington, DC: National Academy Press, Institute of Medicine; 1996.

22. Peek ME, Cargill A, Huang ES. Diabetes health disparities. A systematic review of health care interventions. *Med Care Res Rev.* 2007;64:101S–156S. doi: 10.1177/1077558707305409.

23. U.S. Department of Justice. Title VI of the Civil Rights Act of 1964. http://www.usdoj.gov/crt/cor/coord/titlevi.htm. Accessed, November 28, 2007.

24. Abrahamson JH. *Making Sense of Data.* 2nd ed. New York: Oxford University Press; 1994.

25. Dawson-Saunders B, Trap RG. *Basic and Clinical Biostatistics.* 2nd ed. Norwalk, CT: Appleton & Lange; 1994.

26. Rosenstock IM. Why people use health services. *Milbank Mem Fund Q.* 1996;44:94–124.

27. Rosenstock IM, Strecher VJ, Becker MH. The health belief model and HIV risk behavior change. In: DiClemente RJ, Peterson, JL, eds. *Preventing AIDS: Theories and Methods of Behavioral Interventions.* New York: Plenum Press; 1994:5–24.

28. Fishbein M, Ajzen I. *Belief, Attitude, Intention, and Behavior: An Introduction to Theory and Research.* Reading, MA: Addison-Wesley, 1975. http://people.umass.edu/aizen/f&a1975.html. Accessed December 12, 2008.

29. Ajzen IM. Prediction of goal-directed behavior: attitudes, intentions, and perceived behavioral control. *J Exper Soc Psych.* 1986;22:453–474.

30. Fishbein M, Ajzen I, McArdle J. Changing the behavior of alcoholics: Effects of persuasive communication. In: Ajzen I, Fishbein M, eds. *Understanding Attitudes and Predicting Social Behavior.* Englewood Cliffs, NJ: Prentice-Hall; 1980.

31. Prochaska JO, DiClemente CC. Stages and processes of self-change of smoking: Toward an integrative model of change. *J Consult Clin Psychol.* 1983;51:390–395.

32. Velicer WF, Norman GJ, Fava JL, Prochaska JO. Testing 40 predictions from the Transtheoretical Model. *Addict Behav.* 1999;24:455–469.

33. Prochaska JO, Velicer WF. The transtheoretical model of health behavior change. *Am J Health Prom.* 1997;12:38–48.

34. Bandura A. Perceived self-efficacy in the exercise of control over AIDS infection. In: Mays VM, Albee GW, Schneider SS, eds. *Primary Prevention of AIDS: Psychological Approaches.* Newbury Park, CA: Sage; 1989:128–141.

35. Murray CJ, Kulkarni SC, Ezzati M. Understanding the coronary heart disease versus total cardiovascular mortality paradox: a method to enhance the comparability of cardiovascular death statistics in the United States. *Circulation.* 2006;113:2071–2081.

36. Wilson PWF, D'Agostino RB, Levy D, Belanger AM, Silbershatz H, Kannel WB. Prediction of coronary heart disease using risk factor categories. *Circulation.* 1998;97:1837–1847.

37. Turner ST, Weidman WH, Michels VV, et al. Distribution of sodium-lithium countertransport and blood pressure in Caucasians five to eighty-nine years of age. *Hypertension.* 1989;13:378–391.

38. Labonte R, ed. *Heart Health Inequalities in Canada: Report I.* Ottawa: Health and Welfare, Canada, 1988.

39. Gottlieb B. Using social support to protect and to promote health. *J Primary Prev.* 1987;8:49–70.

40. Bandura A. Self-efficacy mechanism in human agency. *Am J Psychol.* 1982;37: 122–148.

41. Mechanic D. Population health: Challenges for science and society. *Milbank Q.* 2007;85(3):533–559. doi: 10.1111/j.1468-0009.2007.00498.x.

42. Omran AR. 1977. Epidemiologic transition in the U.S.: The health factor in population change. *Popul Bull.* 1977;32:3–41.

43. Wing S. Objectivity and ethics in environmental health science. *Environ Health Perspect.* 2003;11:1809–1818.

44 Jenicek M. Epidemiology, Evidenced-based medicine, and evidence-based public health. *J Epidemiol.* 1997;7:187–197.

45. O'Neall MA, Brownson RC. Teaching evidence-based public health to public health practitioners. *Ann Epidemiol* 2005;15:540–544.

46. Institute of Medicine. *The Future of the Public's Health in the 21st Century.* Washington, DC: National Academies Press; 2002.

INDEX

CPSIA information can be obtained
at www.ICGtesting.com
Printed in the USA
FFOW01n0421230617
37009FF

9 780763 765378